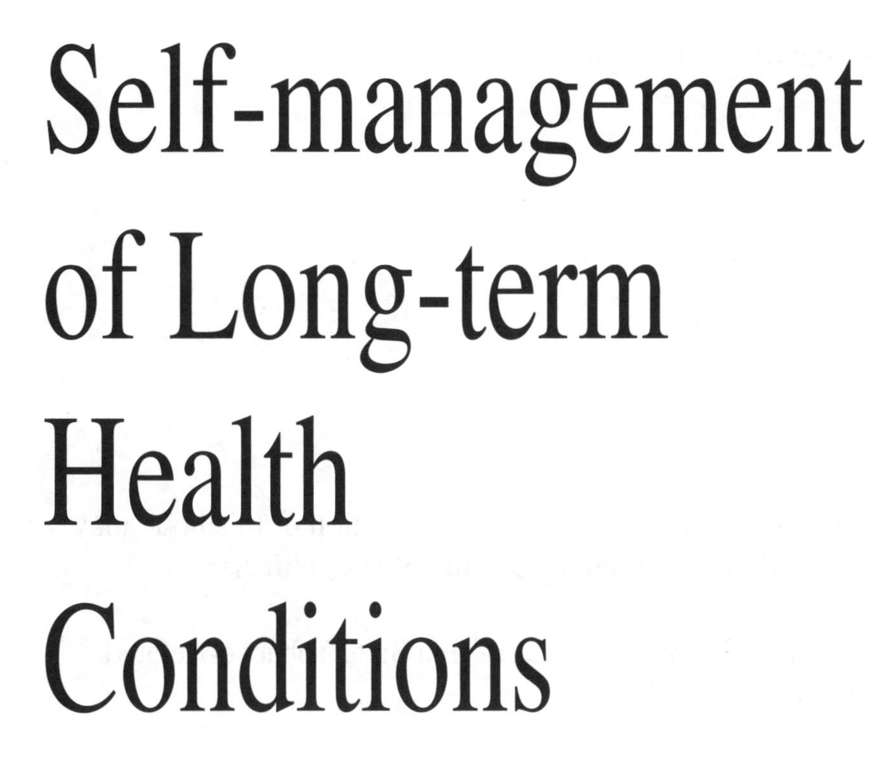

Self-management of Long-term Health Conditions

A Handbook for People with Chronic Disease

Expert Patients Programme Community Interest Company

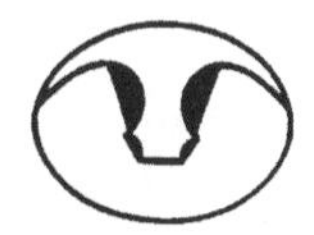

BULL PUBLISHING COMPANY
BOULDER, COLORADO USA

ISBN 978-1-933503-12-7

Bull Publishing Company
P.O. Box 1377
Boulder, Colorado 80306
(303) 545-6350
(303) 545-6354 (fax)
www.bullpub.com

Supported by AHCPR Grant HSO 6680 and California State Tobacco-Related Disease Research Program Award 1RT 156

Publisher: James Bull
Cover Design: Lightbourne Images
Interior Design and Composition: Shadow Canyon Graphics
Illustrations: Publication Services
Editing and Proofreading: see section on Acknowledgments

First Printing

This handbook draws on the material in the US Third Edition of *Living a Healthy Life with Chronic Conditions* by Kate Lorig, Halsted Holman, David Sobel, Diana Laurent, Virginia Gonzalez, Marian Minor and Peg Harrison.

While keeping to the integrity of the US edition, some text has been revised for UK users of the handbook taking into account feedback received since 2002.

Contents

Acknowledgments to the UK Original and Second Editions

Thank you to the many people who have helped compile the original and second editions of this helpbook. In particular, Jim Bull, Kate Lorig, Dr Peter Collins, Jane Cooper, Ayesha Dost, Roy Jones, Anne Kennedy, Dave McHattie, Pete Moore, Brendan O'Rourke, Alison Pollard, Jim Phillips, Dr Vivienne Press, Jean Thompson and Carolyn Townsend. We would also like to thank the many participants and tutors that have given their feedback after attending a self-management course and using the helpbook.

Acknowledgments to the Original US Edition

Many people have helped us write this book. Among the most important are the first 1000 participants of the Stanford University Chronic Disease Self-Management study. These have been followed by thousands of other course participants in the United States, Australia, New Zealand, Canada, and Great Britain. All of these people, along with our wonderful course leaders, have told us what information they needed and helped us make adjustments as we went along.

There are also many professionals who have assisted us: Susan Kayman, Suephy Chen, Sandra Wilson, Margo Harris, Nancy Brannigan, Jim Phillips, Jean Thompson, Lynne Newcombe, John Lynch, Mary Hobbs, Marty Klein, Nazanin Dashtara, Vivian Vestal, María Hernández-Marin, Richard Rubio, and Laurie Doyle. To all of you, your help has been greatly received. A special thanks to Gloria Samuel, who kept us all on track and put this book together.

Finally, thanks to David Bull to whom this book is dedicated. David was our first publisher and had faith in this project that allowed us to proceed. Without him, there may never have been a book. His son Jim has continued the family tradition with support and encouragement for this second edition.

To David Bull,
who made this book possible

Origins of the Expert Patients Programme

'What lies behind us and what lies before us are tiny matters compared to what lies within us.'
— Emerson

A lay-led structured training programme was pioneered by Professor Kate Lorig of Stanford University, California in the 1970s. Her initial practical approach to self-management was enhanced with reference to her colleague Albert Bandura's work on social learning theory. Their first courses were based on the experiences of people living with arthritis.

In the UK Arthritis Care built upon this work and led the way for other organisations to make use of Stanford self-management programmes. In the late 1990's The Long-term Medical Conditions Alliance supported voluntary organisations to deliver courses to people living with a variety of long-term conditions. At the same time the Chief Medical Officer for England set up the Expert Patients Task Force, out of which the Expert Patients Programme (EPP) emerged.

When the first version of this helpbook was published in 2002, the Chief Medical Officer for England, Professor Sir Liam Donaldson, wrote in his introduction:

> "The Expert Patients Programme will help to create a new generation of patients who are empowered to take action in partnership with the health professional caring for them, for example, to reduce pain, to improve the use of medication, and enhance their overall quality of life. Patients will receive the support to help them take more control of their own health and treatment, to make more appropriate use of health and social services, and become more empowered."

In the UK, as elsewhere, lay-led self-management courses have proved to be an effective way of training people with long-term conditions to take an active role in the management of their lives. Since the launch of the EPP in 2002, over 30,000 people living with long-term conditions have attended nearly 3,000 courses run by approximately 1,500 volunteer tutors.

Since 2004 EPP has also led a coalition of organisations across the NHS and voluntary sector to develop Stepping Stones to Quality (SS2Q) a straightforward and practical quality assurance framework. SS2Q is intended for use, in the first instance, by organisations providing Stanford University lay led self-management programmes. In the long term, it is hoped that the values, principles and processes contained in SS2Q will be transferable to all lay led self-management programmes, and that they will be used to support the development of other self-management and self-care interventions.

Five years on, the EPP had demonstrated its worth to such an extent that the Government took steps to facilitate a massive expansion in self-management course places – to 100,000 by the year 2012. To achieve this, it took the bold step of establishing the EPP as the first national Community Interest Company.

The Expert Patients Programme Community Interest Company (EPPCIC) was launched on 1 April 2007. It is a not-for-profit organisation that applies the values of social enterprise to deliver self-management courses, and support other organisations to deliver self-management courses to people living with a wide range of long-term health conditions.

The future EPPCIC will continue to market, support and deliver a range of self-management training courses and services for people living with long-term health conditions. It will increase the number of course places available and increase access among all communities. It will develop new products and services and continue to work in partnership with other providers across the NHS, voluntary sector and social care to ensure equitable provision of lay led self-management across England to all people living with long-term conditions..

August 2007
Expert Patients Programme
Community Interest Company

CHAPTER 1

How to Become an Expert Patient and Active Self-Manager

Nobody wants to have a long-term illness. Unfortunately, many of us will experience chronic illness during our lives. This book has been written to help people with chronic illness to live the healthiest life they can. Perhaps this sounds strange - how can anybody have a long-term illness and live a healthy life at the same time?

This book suggests you can live in a healthy way with a chronic illness, and you do that by working towards overcoming the physical and emotional problems caused by, or associated with, the disease.

The following chapters suggest ways of actively managing your life, with the challenges that accompany a long-term condition. "Active" and "manage" – these are the key words. You can't avoid managing a chronic condition in some way. If you do nothing but suffer, that is a management style. If you only take medication, that is another management style. The book presents a third possibility. You can make a positive choice to be an active self-manager. Actively pursuing your own well-being is a healthy way to live. The book puts forward suggestions for action to support you in your decision to do so.

You will not find any miracles or cures in these pages. There are, certainly, hundreds of tips and ideas to help make your life easier and improve its quality, gathered from doctors, health professionals, and, most importantly, people who have learned to positively manage their illness. But the main purpose of the book is to outline an approach to the active management of some of the problems shared by many people with chronic conditions.

Chronic illness, whatever the specific condition is called, can cause people to lose physical conditioning and to experience fatigue. In addition, it may cause emotional distress such as frustration, anger, depression, or a sense of helplessness. Active managers step outside the immediate difficulty of their situation, to take an overview of their life. They explore what they might do to minimise their symptoms and the effects of their condition. They decide to promote their own health. Health is not just absence of disease. It is soundness of mind and body, and a healthy life is one that seeks that soundness. Active managers aim to create a sound healthy basis for a life of the greatest possible physical capability and optimum happiness.

As an active self-manager, you play the central role in your healthy life, chronic condition and all. You take control of your life and that is a very healthy thing to do.

What Is A Chronic Condition?

Health problems can be described as "acute" or "chronic."

Acute health problems usually begin abruptly, have a single, easily diagnosed cause, are of short duration and will respond to a specific treatment, such as medication or surgery. For most acute illnesses, a cure with a return to normal health is expected. For the patient and the doctor there is relatively little uncertainty; both usually know what to expect. The illness typically gets worse for a while, is treated, and then gets better. Appendicitis is an example of an acute illness. It begins suddenly, signalled by nausea and pain in the abdomen. The diagnosis of appendicitis, established by physical examination, leads to surgery for removal of the inflamed appendix. There follows a period of recovery and then a return to normal health. A health professional can usually manage the care of their patient over a relatively short space of time by finding and administering effective treatment

Chronic illnesses are different. They begin slowly and proceed slowly. Arthritis, for example, generally starts with brief annoying twinges that gradually increase. Unlike acute disease, chronic illnesses have multiple causes that vary over time and include heredity, lifestyle factors such as smoking, lack of exercise, poor diet and stress, and exposure to harmful environmental influences. Managing a chronic illness can be frustrating for anyone who, naturally, wants a quick solution. It is difficult for the doctor and the patient when immediate answers aren't available. In some cases, even when diagnosis is rapid, as in the case of a stroke or heart attack, the course and long-term effects of the illness may be hard to predict. The absence of a regular or predictable pattern is a major characteristic of most chronic illnesses.

Symptoms Are Inter-Related

Unlike acute disease, where full recovery is expected, chronic illness often leads over time to more symptoms and loss of physical functioning. Many people assume that the symptoms they are experiencing are due to only one cause: the disease. While a disease can certainly cause pain, shortness of breath, fatigue and so on, it is not the only cause. Each symptom can by itself contribute to other symptoms, and all of them together can make each single one worse. Symptoms can feed on each other. For example, depression causes fatigue, stress causes tense muscles, leading to more pain or shortness of breath, and so on. The interactions of these symptoms, in turn, make the condition worse. It can become a vicious cycle that deteriorates unless the cycle is broken. (see Figure 1.1)

This book examines ways of breaking the cycle and solving the problems of physical and emotional helplessness which can result from chronic illness.

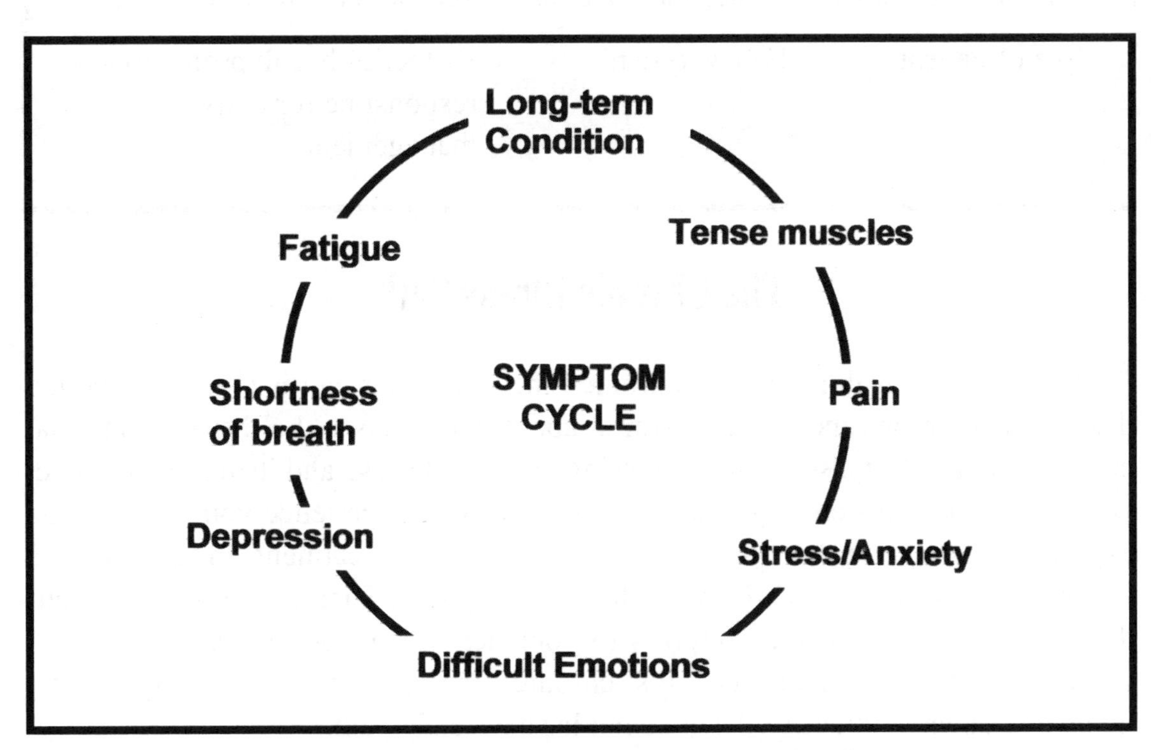

Figure 1.1 *The Vicious Symptom Circle*

Table 1.1 *Differences Between Acute and Chronic Disease*

	Acute Disease	**Chronic Disease (long-term)**
Beginning	Rapid	Gradual
Cause	Usually one	Many
Duration	Short	Indefinite
Diagnosis	Commonly accurate	Often uncertain, especially early on
Diagnostic Tests	Often decisive	Often of limited value
Treatment	Cure common	Cure rare
Role of Professional	Select and conduct	Teacher and therapy partner
Role of Patient	Follow orders	Partner of health professionals, responsible for daily management

The Chronic Illness Path

The first responsibility of any chronic illness self-manager is to understand the disease. This means more than learning about what causes the disease and what can be done for it. It also means observing how the disease and its treatment affect you. A disease is different for each person, and with experience you will become expert at determining the effects of the disease and its treatment. In fact, you are the only person who lives with your disease every day. Therefore, observing your disease and making accurate reports to your health care providers are essential parts of being a good manager. Most chronic illnesses and associated symptoms go up and down in intensity. They do not have a steady path.

The visits on the graph in Figure 1.2 represent Pat's regular follow-up appointments with the doctor or other health professional. Even though the intensity of Pat's symptoms is at the same level for all three visits, what has happened in the time between appointments can mean entirely different things when the health care team is evaluating whether to maintain or change treatment. In the case of the first visit, the symptoms are getting better, so keeping the treatment stable or even

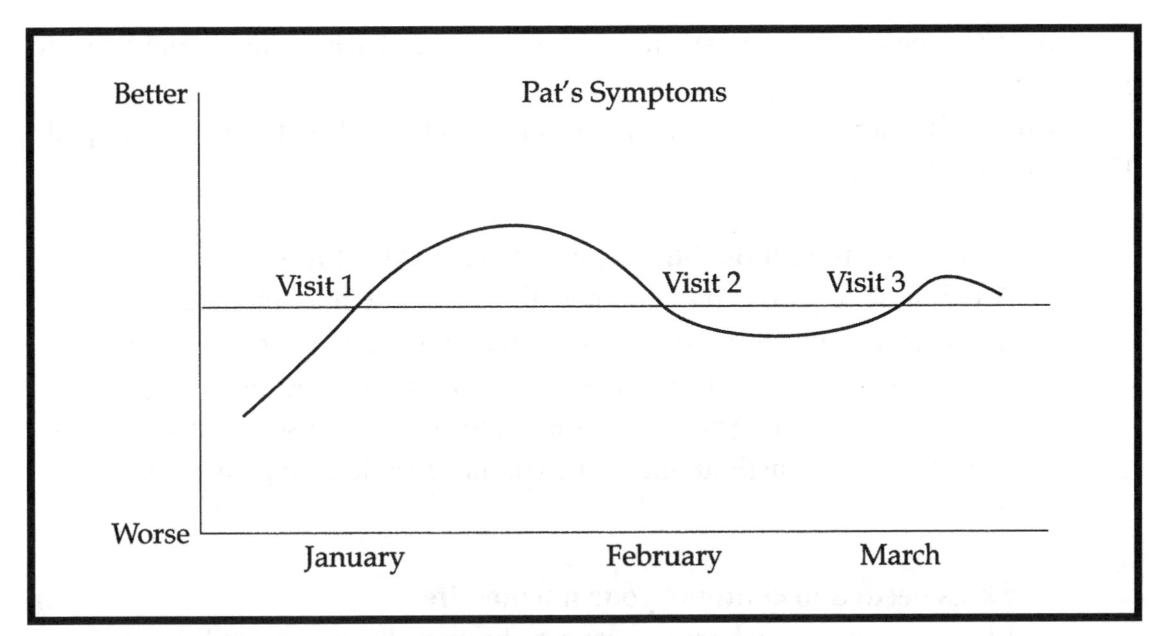

Figure 1.2 *Illness Path*

lessening it may be in order. In the case of the second visit, things seem to be getting worse, so additional treatment may be the choice. In the case of the third visit, things have been stable for a while, so maintaining treatment may be the best treatment option.

Everyday Self-Management Skills

All chronic illnesses need day-to-day management.
The key to success is:

- deciding what you want to do
- deciding how you are going to do it
- practising regularly what works for you

What you do about something depends on how you think about it. The thoughts you have can greatly influence how you cope with your health related problems. More about this in chapter 5. Some of the most successful self-managers think of their illness as a path. The path goes up and down. Sometimes it is flat and smooth, other times it is rough. Sometimes you can go quickly, other times you must slow down. Sometimes, particularly steep hills mean you might have to put more work in, other times, you might be able to get away with working less hard. There may be obstacles on your path and you have to find ways to get around them.

Good self-managers have learned the skills they need to travel on the path. These skills fall into three main categories:

- **Skills to deal with the illness and manage symptoms**
  Any illness requires you to do new things. These may include taking medicine, checking your symptoms, or using oxygen. It means more frequent interactions with your doctor and the health and social care system. Sometimes there are new exercises or a new diet. All these constitute the work you need to do to manage your illness.

- **Skills needed to continue your normal life**
  Life goes on even when you have a chronic illness. You still have housework, friendships to keep up, jobs to manage and family relationships to keep going. Things that you once took for granted can become much more complicated in the face of chronic illness. You may need to learn new skills to carry on with your daily activities so that you can go on enjoying life. Sometimes, you may need to really look at some of the things you are doing and ask whether doing them differently might work better.

- **Skills needed to deal with emotions**
  When you are diagnosed as having a chronic illness, your plans for your future may have to change and changes can lead to negative emotions. They may include: anger—'Why me? It's not fair'; depression—'I can't do anything any more, what's the use'; frustration—'No matter what I do it doesn't make any difference'; or isolation—'No one understands, no one wants to be around someone who is ill.' Dealing with these negative emotions is a skill you can learn.

With this as background, you can think of self-management as the use of skills to

1. manage the work of dealing with your illness,
2. manage the work of continuing your daily activities, and
3. manage the changing emotions brought about by chronic illness.

Self-Management Tasks

1. **take care of your illness**
2. **carry out your normal activities**
3. **manage your emotional changes**

Throughout this book you will find information to help you learn and practise self-management skills. This is not a textbook. You don't need to read every word in every chapter. Instead, read the first two chapters and then use the table of contents to find the information you need. Feel free to skip around. In this way you will learn the skills you need to negotiate your individual path.

No matter what long-term health condition you have, you can use your own skills, imagination and information sources to manage your life better.

• • •

Suggested Further Reading

Campling, Frankie. *Living with a Long-term Illness* (Facts). Oxford: Oxford University Press, 2006.

Donoghue, Paul J. and Siegel, Mary E. *Sick and Tired of Feeling Sick and Tired: Living with Invisible Chronic Illness*. London: WW Norton & Company Ltd., 2000.

Sobel, David., and Robert Ornstein. *The Healthy Mind, Healthy Body Handbook*. Feltham.: Time Life UK, 1998.

Sobel, David, and Robert Ornstein. *Healthy Pleasures*, 2nd ed. Reading, Mass.: Addison-Wesley, 1997.

Sobel, David., and Robert Ornstein. *Mind & Body Health Handbook: How to Use Your Mind & Body to Relieve Stress, Overcome Illness, and Enjoy Healthy Pleasures*, 2nd ed. Feltham: Time Life UK, 1998.

CHAPTER 2

Becoming an Active Self-Manager

How do you eat an elephant?
One bite at a time.

You can't avoid being a self-manager if you have a chronic condition. Some people manage themselves by withdrawing from life. They socialise less, they stay in the house, they even stay in bed. The condition becomes their life. Other people with the same condition and symptoms manage by getting on with their life. They may have to change what they do or the way they do it, but their life continues to be full and active. The difference between these two extremes is not the disease but the decision. Becoming a more active self-manager involves making choices. It's up to you to decide what you want to do.

This book is intended to help you carry through your decision to be active, healthier and happier. Active self-management is a skill and like any skill, it can be learned. You get better at it as you go along. You see increasingly how you can use it in many situations. This chapter will start you on your way.

You are your own manager.

Action Planning (or One Bite at a Time)

The following seven steps are good self- management practice, which will help you to take charge of your life.

1. decide what you want to achieve

2. look for alternative ways to achieve this goal
3. make a short-term action plan
4. carry out your action plan
5. check your results
6. make changes as needed
7. reward yourself

The seven steps in more detail in a moment, but first, here's an example.

Deciding what you want to achieve may involve exploring feelings first. Rushing this stage may leave underlying feelings or desires unexplored, so take time to notice what goes on in your mind as you formulate what you want to do. Let's say you are unhappy but not sure why. Thinking about it more, you find you miss contact with an old friend who has moved. You realise it would make you happy to see this friend. Having worked out what you want, you decide to go. Immediately, you are aware of a large number of problems, but still, you do now have your goal clear.

Travelling raises a lot of problems in your mind, but you take them one by one and see what you might do about them. In the past you have always driven, but you find it tiring, so you look for other ways. You consider leaving at noon instead of early in the morning and making the journey in two days instead of one. You consider asking a friend along to share the driving. A coach is possible, but the coach station is some distance from your friend's house. There is also a train that goes within ten miles of your destination. That might be more expensive than you can easily manage, but with off-peak fares and booking in advance, the cost can be kept down. You decide to take the train.

The trip still seems overwhelming, as there is so much to prepare. You decide to write down all the steps necessary to make the visit a reality. These include finding a good time to go, buying a ticket, working out how to pack the minimum and handle your luggage, seeing if you can make it up and down the stairs to the train, wondering if you can walk on a moving train to get food or find the toilet, and sorting out how you will get to the station.

You start by making an action plan. In the short-term, that is, this week, you will ring up to find out just how much the train company can help. You also decide to start taking a short walk each day and walking up and down a few steps so that you can be steadier on your feet and feel more confident in walking. So you carry out your action plan by phoning the train company and starting your walking programme.

A week later you check the results. Looking back at all the difficulties you had to work through, you find that a single telephone call answered many questions.

The train staff are used to people who have mobility problems and they have settled many of your worries. However, you are still concerned about walking. Even though you are walking better, you are still unsteady and uncertain. You make a change in your plan by asking a physiotherapist about this, and she suggests using a walking-stick. Although you hate it, you find that a stick gives you that extra security needed on a moving train.

Now you are ready to make a new action plan for accomplishing some of the other tasks necessary to make the journey possible. What once seemed like a dream is becoming a reality.

At this point, you may like to consider adopting a notebook as a self-management journal. The topics covered in this book can be considered independently of each other, but quite often there are overlaps – naturally, because the topics are all concerned with managing your daily life. The basis of the method discussed in this chapter is to formulate your current thoughts and habits and problems into words, and to write them down so you can see them and think about them, and review them later. Some of the information you gather and the thinking you do can be of use for other topics. A shorter alternative might be to log events in a word or two on a calendar or in a diary.

Some people write down their symptoms in the diary, so that they can work out whether certain activities or moods are making the symptoms worse. Others find that writing down symptom levels tends to concentrate the mind on the symptoms, so they can appear worse. You might want to work out for yourself whether writing down symptom levels is right for you.

The seven self-managements steps in detail are the backbone of any self-management programme. You will be able to apply these, maybe adapted a little, to other areas of your life as discussed in later chapters of this book.

The Seven Self-Management Steps

1. Deciding What You Want To Achieve

The first step is to decide on your goal.

This may be the most difficult step. Be realistic and very specific. Think of all the things you would like to do. Importantly, try to make sure the goal is one that is right for you and not one that you feel you need to achieve in order to satisfy other people in your life.

One example is a woman who wanted to climb twenty steps to her daughter's home so that she could join her family for a special meal. Another person wanted to lose weight to help his cardiac condition. Someone else wanted to get out and do more but felt limited by having to take her oxygen tank everywhere. In each case, the goal was one that would take several weeks or even months to accomplish.

Perhaps you feel uncertain about what may be considered a realistic goal, for example, to decide how many steps to climb. In such a situation you may wish to set a goal after discussing it with a chosen "consultant" – someone you choose to talk to. It could be your doctor or other health and social care professionals.

One of the problems with goals is that they may often seem like dreams, so unlikely that we don't even try to tackle them. For now, take a moment to write down your goals, either in your journal or here. Don't worry about what you learned as a child—it is all right to write in your own book!

Goals:

1. ____

2. ____

3. ____

Put a star (★) against the goal you would like to work on first.

2. Looking For Alternative Ways to Achieve Your Goal

The second step a self-manager will take is to think around the possible routes to a goal.

Sometimes, what stops us reaching our goal is not that it is too far off, or just a dream—it is simply that we do not see or think about the various ways to reach any specified goal. In the earlier example, the traveller who wanted to visit a friend made a list of alternative ways of travelling before opting for the train. The mother who wanted to climb twenty steps could start off with a slow walking programme, or she could climb up and down a few steps each day, or she could look into having the special family meal at a different place. The man who wanted to lose weight could decide not to eat between meals or to give up desserts, or start an exercise programme. The woman who wanted to do more outside her home could find out about courses at a local Further Education College, or contact friends by phone or letter or email.

The people in these examples had more than one option open to them. Your self-manager's job here is to list all the options you can think of for reaching your selected goal. Then choose one or two to work with. If it's hard to think of lots of different options by yourself, now's the time to consult your family, friends or health care professionals. Other consultants at this stage could be people in your community such as work colleagues or local club, charity or religious leaders. The Internet might provide useful ideas as well. When you approach your consultants, don't ask what you should do. Instead, ask for suggestions. Add the suggestions to your list of options.

Don't assume that a choice doesn't exist or won't work until you have properly looked into it. There is always something you haven't thought of. For example, a woman who had lived in the same town her whole life was having trouble arranging for transport to hospital. A friend suggested a voluntary car scheme. The woman said there was no such service where she lived. It was only when her friend came to visit and rang a local agency that she learnt the town had three voluntary schemes and one Council run service that could help her. So, never assume anything.

Either take your self-management journal, or use the spaces below, to write down a list of the options open to you to reach your main goal. Decide which two or three you would like to try.

Options

1. ______________________________

2. ______________________________

3. ______________________________

4. ______________________________

3. Making Short-Term Plans—Action Planning

The third step is to turn your options into short-term plans. These are action plans.

You are planning for actions you know you will be able to take in the next week. You are, in a way, making an agreement with yourself to take steps towards the goal you have identified. The action plan should be about something you want to get done. You make an action plan as a tool to help you do what you wish, not to please your friends, family or doctor.

Action plans are probably your most important self-management tool. Most of us can do things to make us healthier, but fail to do them. For example, most people with a chronic illness can walk, some just across the room, others can walk a mile or so. However, few people have a systematic exercise programme based on considered action plans.

An action plan will help you do the things you know you want to do. Working through the steps to a realistic action plan is an important skill that may well determine the success of your self-management programme. A realistic action plan is one that helps you become more confident and therefore able to do more over time. An unrealistic action plan is one where you 'overreach' yourself and lose confidence.

Making Your Action Plan

1. **Decide what you will do to move towards your goal this week.**
   A step-climber might decide to climb three steps once a day for four days. A man trying to lose weight may decide not to eat between meals for three days and to walk round the block before dinner on the following four days. You may want to consult with your health and social care professionals, to give you confidence that what you want to do is realistic and a step on the way to your long-term goal.

2. **Make sure your plan states what you will actually do.**
   Rather than decide "to relax", decide, 'I will listen to my progressive muscle relaxation tape.'

3. **Plan in detail.**
   a. Exactly what are you going to do? How far will you walk? How will you eat less? What breathing technique will you practise?

b. How much will you do? Will you walk for 15 minutes? Not eat between meals for three days? Practise breathing exercises for 15 minutes?
c. When will you do this? Before lunch? In the shower? When you come home from work? Connecting a new activity to an old habit is a good way to make sure it gets done. Another trick is to do your new activity before an old favourite such as reading the newspaper or a TV programme you always watch.
d. How often will you do the activity? We would all like to do things every day, but it is not always possible. It is usually best to decide to do something three or four times a week. If you do more, so much the better. However, if you are like most of us, you will feel less pressure if you can do your activity three or four times and still be successful at your action plan.

Please note! Taking medications is an exception. This must be done exactly as decided together with your doctor.

4. **Start planning from where you are and plan to start slowly.** If you can walk for one minute, plan to start your walking programme by walking one minute once every hour or two, not by walking a mile. If you have never done any exercise, start with a few minutes of warm-up. A total of five or ten minutes is enough. If you want to lose weight, set a goal based on your existing eating habits, such as not eating after dinner. "Losing a pound this week" is not an action plan. "Eat nothing after dinner" sets out what you will actually do.

5. **Give yourself some time off.** All people have days when they don't feel like doing anything. That is a good reason for saying that you will do something three times a week instead of every day. In this way, if you don't feel like walking one day, you can still achieve your action plan. Pace yourself.

6. **Once you've made your action plan, ask yourself the following question:** "On a scale of 0 to 10, with 0 being totally unsure and 10 being totally certain, how certain am I that I can complete this plan?" If your answer is 7 or above, this is probably a realistic

A Successful Action Plan:

1. **Is something YOU want to do**
2. **Is achievable**
3. **Is linked to specific behaviour**
4. **Answers the questions**
   What?
   How much?
   When?
   How often?
5. **Is something you are confident you can achieve**

action plan. Congratulate yourself; you have done the hard work. If your answer is below 7, then you should look again at your action plan. Ask yourself why you're not confident. What problems do you foresee? Then see if you can either solve the problems or change your plan to make yourself more confident of success.

7. **When you have made a plan you are happy with, write it out clearly and put it where you will see it every day.**
   Keep track of how you are doing and the problems you encounter. Page 19 is a completed example of an action plan. Pages 20 and 21 are blanks; make copies of them to use weekly, or use the format in your self-management journal.

4. Carrying Out Your Action Plan

The fourth step, of course, is to do it!

A well thought-out, realistic plan is easy to follow. Ask your family or friends to check on how you are doing - telling them about your progress will keep you motivated. Keep track of your daily activities while carrying out your plan. All good managers have lists of what they want to accomplish. Tick things off on your chart or in your diary when you finish doing them. Make notes of any problems you have. This will give you guidance on how realistic your planning was and will also be useful in making future plans. The notes will help you see if there is a pattern to any problems and increase your skill at problem-solving. For example, the woman who wanted to increase her stair-climbing capacity never did her climbing. Each day she had a different problem; not enough time, being tired, the weather being too cold, and so on. When she looked back at her notes, she began to realise that the real problem was her fear of falling with no-one around to help her. She then decided to use a stick while climbing stairs, and to do it when a friend or neighbour was around.

5. Check Your Results

The fifth step, at the end of each week, is to see how much of your action plan you have carried out.

Think about how near you are to reaching your goal. Are you able to walk farther? Have you lost weight? Are you less fatigued? Taking stock is important. You may not see progress day by day, but you should see a little progress each week. At the end of each week, check on how well you have fulfilled your action plan.

If you are having problems, this is the time to problem-solve.

6. Make Changes—Solve Problems

The sixth step is necessary if, as is often the case, the first plan is not the most workable.

If there are difficulties with it, don't give up. Try something else to solve your problem. Change your short-term plans so that your steps are easier, give yourself more time, choose new steps towards your goal, get more advice from your consultants or help from other people. Work out what the real problem is. For example: you know the stairs are difficult, but it takes a bit more thought to work out that your real problem is a fear of falling. Make a list of ideas to solve that. Maybe ask other people to help you with this. Pick one idea to try. Remember that new activities are often difficult. Think about how successful you have been, when you've given your idea a chance to work. If you still have the problem, try another of your ideas.

Sometimes you may have to accept that your problem is not solvable now. This can be hard to do. It doesn't mean, though, that it won't be solvable later. Even if your path seems completely blocked, there are probably alternative paths. You can try again in a while. Don't give up. Keep going.

Summary of Problem-Solving Steps

1. **Identify the problem**
2. **List ideas to solve the problem**
3. **Select one method to try**
4. **Assess the results**
5. **Try another idea if the first didn't work**
6. **Use other resources**
7. **Accept that the problem may not be solvable now**

7. Rewarding Yourself

The seventh step involves one big reward and a lot of little ones.

The big reward for being a good self-manager comes from achieving your goals and living a fuller and more comfortable life.

The little ones are what you award yourself by setting simple and easy goals and rewarding yourself often. Perhaps you won't read the paper until after your exercise so that reading the paper becomes your reward. Maybe you spend the money you have saved by stopping smoking on fruit or on an outing. Rewards don't have to be expensive or fattening! There are many healthy pleasures that can add enjoyment to your life.

Summary of Successful Self-Management Steps

1. **Sets goals**
2. **Makes a list of alternatives for reaching the goal**
3. **Makes short-term action plans toward that goal**
4. **Carries out the plan**
5. **Checks on progress weekly**
6. **Makes changes to deal with new problems on the way**
7. **Uses rewards for a job well done**

Example of a completed Action Plan

When you write your action plan, be sure it includes:

1. what you are going to do
2. how much you are going to do
3. when you are going to do it
4. how many days a week you are going to do it

For example:
This week ……
what: I will walk around the block
how much: twice
when: before lunch
how many: three days this week.
How confident are you that you can complete this plan?
(0= not at all confident; 10= totally confident)
Record your score here: _____9_____

	Tick	**Comments**
Monday	—	Raining
Tuesday	3	Walked slowly & noticed everything around me
Wednesday	3	It was cool out, but the walk felt good
Thursday	—	Raining again
Friday	3	Only walked around the block once
Saturday	3	Took a friend along, we talked about the neighbours
Sunday	—	Felt tired
Overall Comment		Exceeded my expectations and walked around the block four days this week.

Record your comments on how your plan went

Action Plan

This week ……
what:
how much:
when:
how many:
How confident are you that you can complete this plan?
(0= not at all confident; 10= totally confident)
Record your score here: _________

	Tick	Comments
Monday		
Tuesday		
Wednesday		
Thursday		
Friday		
Saturday		
Sunday		
Overall Comment		

Record your comments on how your plan went

Action Plan

This week ......
what:
how much:
when:
how many:
How confident are you that you can complete this plan?
(0= not at all confident; 10= totally confident)
Record your score here: _________

	Tick	**Comments**
Monday		
Tuesday		
Wednesday		
Thursday		
Friday		
Saturday		
Sunday		
Overall Comment		

Record your comments on how your plan went

It is, obviously, true that not all goals are achievable. Chronic illness may mean having to reappraise or give up some options. If this is true for you, notice properly that you are sorry that you can't do everything you want, and then move on. There are some suggestions in chapter 15 Planning for the Future for dealing with loss, but in general don't spend energy on what you can't do—instead start work on another goal you would like to achieve. Focus on all the things you can do and enjoy them to the fullest.

This book is intended to support you in your intention to manage life with your long-term condition yourself. Most self-management skills are similar for all conditions. The rest of the book discusses approaches to various aspects of life as a self-manager: finding resources; symptom management including using your mind; exercise; communicating; sex and intimacy; making clear your wishes about future health care; healthy eating; managing your medicines and making treatment decisions, dealing with the future, and many tips and hints for making life easier. You can skip around the chapters depending on the information you are looking for—use the table of contents or the index at the back, or you can read right through the book.

• • •

Suggested Further Reading

Baker, Barbara. *Coping with Long Term Illness (Overcoming Common Problems)* London: Sheldon Press, 2001.

Lorig, Kate and James Fries. *The Arthritis Self Help Book.* 5th Edition, Addison-Wesley, 2001.

Milstrey Wells, S. *A Delicate Balance: Living Successfully with Chronic Illness.* Perseus Books Group, 2000.

Sobel, David and Robert Ornstein. *Healthy Pleasures.* 2nd ed. Mass: Addison-Wesley, 1997.

CHAPTER
3

Finding Resources

Its not what you know, it's who you know (and can consult).

To be the successful self-manager of your life with a chronic condition, you'll need to know when you could use some help and how to find it. Getting help with parts of your life does not mean that you are victim to your illness nor that you are weak. Knowing where to go for help takes initiative, strength, energy and good organisation. It will be necessary to evaluate your condition and your own capabilities as you work out what you want to do, and use the seven self-management steps towards achieving it.

If you find a problem difficult to solve on your own, part of your action plan may be to seek something or someone to help you. You can weigh up objectively what help from elsewhere will enable you to do the things you want. Then use the first major resource in your life—other people. You can get information of huge value from talking to other people. Calling these people "consultants" shows the sort of relationship to seek. In all areas of self-management, yours is the final decision, but the answers you get from those you consult can feed into your list of options at stage 2 of any action plan. A consultant is someone trustworthy that you can talk to confidently about your condition; it could be a doctor, but it might just as easily be anyone else in your life. Gradually, you will build up a network of consultants.

An option when you seek a consultant is to "use" your family or friends. You may possibly ask them directly for help. This can be hard. In chapter 9 Communicating there is a discussion of how to choose the right words to ask for help. However, most people—family or no—want to help, but don't know how until you ask them, so your job is to learn how to ask for help and tell them clearly what you need.

Another option, if you live on your own or if asking is too difficult, is to look for other resources in your community. These may be tradespeople, like carpenters, or professionals, like accountants, or a man with a van. They may be organisations like the Citizens' Advice Bureau or an electrical shop with a person who comes out to fix washing machines. They may be places where information is stored, like the public library. Identifying resources round where you live can be a bit like a treasure hunt. It may be as simple as looking in the telephone book and making some calls, or using the Internet. Or it may take more effort and thought. Use an action plan to keep your goals clear and explore the options systematically, including starting all over again at the problem-solving stage when a clue doesn't lead to treasure!

Perhaps the problem you identify is that you get irritable preparing an evening meal. As in the example in chapter 2 of the woman who did not practise her stair-climbing, you realise you don't hate cooking, it's just that you can't stand up for very long. Your goal is to keep on cooking for yourself. So you must explore the options – one of which is getting your kitchen altered so you can prepare meals sitting down. Hunting out resources is part of information gathering stage of action planning.

You start by talking to other people who may remember someone who has had similar work done. You could find out a lot about costs and problems from them. You might look in the yellow pages for builders or architects. Some of them specialise in kitchens, but maybe none mentions anything about designing for people with physical limitations. You plan to make a couple of phone calls. You do so but have to go back to the options when you can't find anyone with the right experience in design.

So what other options are open? You could look for names in the local paper or see if anyone has advertised their details at the local post office or the corner shop. Perhaps contact the Occupational Therapist in your local social services department. Explore the databases in your library reference section. The Citizens' Advice Bureau has a resource database. You could also seek support at your regular place of worship.

There are some people in every community who seem to know who is who and where everything is. They can be useful consultants. They tend to be people who have been living there a long time and who have got involved in the community. They could be a friend, a person who runs a local club, a religious leader of any faith, a doctor or school secretary, a librarian, the postman, or someone who works at the local newsagents. It's worth asking someone like this – and once you get good at thinking about and using your community resources, you will soon find that other people start to consult you too.

You have probably done this sort of hunting many times. The difference now is that you do it systematically and within a time frame. Your action plan will have in it tasks for the next week, so you do your resource-hunting in steps you can manage in a few days. What's more, you will probably be keeping a record of what you've done and the information you've gathered. Next time you will have the beginnings of a large support network already in place.

Resources for Resources

When you need to find goods or services, there are some resources you can call on to find more resources.

Some examples are:

- The telephone directory — the business pages of the local BT Phonebook, Yellow Pages or the Thompson Directory
- Your local library
- Disabled Living Centre or Independent Living Centre which keep up-to-date catalogues of equipment for people with any form of physical problem
- Shops and Pharmacies supplying medical equipment
- Council for Voluntary Service or Rural Community Council
- National Council for Voluntary Organisations
- Voluntary groups concerned with particular long-term conditions—if you can't find a local branch, find their national office
- There are a large number of telephone helpline services now available from the Internet or your local library will be able to get you a list. Health and social care related voluntary agencies dedicated to a disease may have a helpline, such as Arthritis Care, BACUP (cancer), Diabetes UK, the National Asthma Campaign, the British Heart Foundation, or the Multiple Sclerosis Society.

Patient support organisations provide up-to-date information about your disease and advice, plus guidance and support on daily living issues. Many of them fund research that they hope will help people live better with their disease and may lead to a cure. They will send you newsletters and information leaflets on request; for a membership fee, you can also join these organisations.

Most patient support organisations have good Internet websites. See the end of the chapter for listings.

NHS Choices is a really good website that can help you find out more about your specific medical condition.

Financial Matters

Citizens' Advice Bureaus, Law Centres and Independent Welfare Rights groups, usually affiliated to the Federation of Independent Advice Centres FIAC, are good places to visit to find out about state benefits or financial matters. Some Social Services Departments in cities also offer these services. Some will make home visits to help you sort out problems. Any government benefit agency only has to provide you with accurate information, it does not have to advise you in your best interests. It is a good idea to use independent agencies to get a full review of the benefits you are entitled to.

Other Organisations

There are other types of organisations which may be of help to you. Some of these are:

- Ex-military organisations if you or a close relative have been in the forces. The Royal British Legion or the Soldiers, Sailors and Airman's Families Association (SSAFA) can give you information.
- Religious organisations. Many religious organisations have advisory services. You do not need to be a member of a religious organisation to receive help. Local Parishes, Diocese, The Salvation Army, Mosques, Temples or Gurdwaras, for example, have good information about local services.
- Domestic violence organisations. Domestic violence against people with chronic disease can happen. Local refuges treat all enquiries seriously and in confidence. Their addresses are not made public but they can be contacted through the local police or social services.
- Local authority services. Housing Advice Centres can help you find somewhere to live or find grants to improve things such as heating and insulation. Social services have a duty to provide advice

for disabled people. The advice is free, but you have to buy, or contribute towards, any equipment you may need. There may be grants that you can apply for if you do not have adequate resources.

- Disability Employment Advisors (DEA) are attached to Job Centres run by the employment agency. They can help you if you are working and have a chronic condition or disability that will last for more than six months. They can also help if you are planning to get back to work. The Disability Discrimination Act gives you real protection and can help to make sure your employer is able to find ways to keep you employed by providing special equipment or facilities. Do not think about resigning from your job on the grounds of ill health until you have talked to a DEA.
- NHS Direct is a telephone and website service run mainly by nurses who can give health-related information. They can give you advice over the phone (0845 4647) or can suggest what you should do next.
- Local Librarians can help you use the computer databases and reference section of a library. Make sure that any medical or health-related books you use to get information have been published very recently as a specific treatment may have changed. Librarians will know about specialist libraries not open to the public and can order books and journals for you from anywhere in the country. For a small fee, you can order copies of articles published in journals. You may be able to get access to a university medical library which will have a wide collection of books and journals. Medical books may contain information in great detail. Use the information of interest or relevance to you. You may find details about helpful organisations at the back of books, and there will also be reading lists and bibliographies at the end for more sources of information.
- Government documents can be bought through HMSO (Her Majesty's Stationery Office) or they can be downloaded from government websites for free.
- Local and national newspapers sometimes have a health editor who may have a file of information or may even be interested in helping you to track down something you want to read. In relevant sections of newspapers, local organisations advertise classes, lectures and meetings that you could attend.

The Internet

The fastest-growing resource in our society today is the Internet. Information is being added to this worldwide network at a dizzying rate every day, every second. The Internet, all electronic information transfer, including e-mail and graphical Web pages, and the World Wide Web, the graphical interface to the Internet that we are most familiar with, offer not only a nearly endless supply of information about health and anything else you can imagine, but also opportunities to interact with people all over the world. Someone who has a rare health condition might find it difficult to find others with the same disease where they live. With the Internet, though, there might be a whole group of such people to talk to - it doesn't matter whether they are across the street or on the other side of the world.

The good thing about the Internet is that anyone can have a Web site. The bad thing about the Internet is that anyone can have a Web site. The Internet has virtually no controls over who is posting information or whether the information is correct, or even safe. This can mean that there is a lot of information out there that might be very useful, because individuals can share it quickly. It can also mean that someone might post incorrect or dangerous information. Don't assume that information found on the Internet is true. Approach the information with scepticism and caution: Is the author or the sponsor of the Web site clearly identified? Is the author reputable? Is the information contrary to what everyone else seems to be saying about the subject? Does common sense support the information? What is the purpose of the Web site? Are they trying to sell you something?

Study the Website address, the URL (Uniform Resource Locator), which starts with http://. For example, the Department of Health website is: http://www.doh.gov.uk/

http:// means 'hyper text transfer protocol.' 'www' means that the website is on the World Wide Web. 'dh' is short for Department of Health. 'gov' means that the website is a government site. 'uk' means that the site has originated in the UK.

You will often see .edu, .org, .gov or .com as part of a website's URL. If there are no initials for a country (such as uk) at the end of a URL, it means the website is probably based in the USA.

In the UK, URLs ending with .ac.uk indicate that it is an academic institution.

Private, voluntary organisations and 'not-for-profit' organisations have .org.uk at the end. Private companies in the UK also may have .co.uk at the end.

If you want to try using the web for the first time, many libraries now have computers which you can use for a small fee or you could try an Internet Café. If you think you might use the Internet a great deal on your home computer, look out for special Internet connection packages to avoid huge telephone bills.

Here are some examples of useful health-related websites in the UK

NHS Choices
www.nhs.uk
Offers a comprehensive website with really good information about most health conditions

NHS Direct
www.nhsdirect.nhs.uk
Access to Care Website provides an understanding about the issues affecting access to health care services in the UK
http://www.his.path.cam.ac.uk/phealth/access/access.htm

BBC health
http://www.bbc.co.uk/health/
What should I do? describes a number of commonly occurring health problems and provides advice about what you can do yourself
http://www.whatshouldido.com/

DIPEx is the world's first Database of Individual Patient Experiences in Hypertension, Prostate and Breast Cancer
http://www.dipex.org/

British Medical Journal
http://www.bmj.com/index.shtml
Information on BSE
http://www.cjd.ed.ac.uk

OMNI (Organizing Medical Networked Information) is a gateway to Internet resources in medicine, and health care
http://omni.nott.ac.uk

Public Health Genetics Unit provides news and information about advances in genetics and their impact on prevention of disease
http://www.medinfo.cam.ac.uk/phgu/default.asp

Disabled Living Foundation
www.dlf.org.uk

Patient UK is a directory of health, disease and related websites from the UK
www.patient.co.uk

Age Concern
www.ageconcern.org.uk

Arthritis Care
www.arthritiscare.org.uk

British Heart Foundation
www.bhf.org.uk

Diabetes UK
www.diabetes.org.uk

Multiple Sclerosis Society
www.mssociety.org.uk

Femail netdoctor has good information on medicines; it is the medical section of the Daily Mail's women's section
http://femail.netdoctor.co.uk

CHAPTER 4

Understanding and Managing Common Symptoms

You are the expert on you.

Chronic illnesses come with symptoms. Specific diseases tend to have identifying symptoms, but people with various long-term conditions often have symptoms in common. This chapter looks at managing some of those common symptoms.

Symptoms are information to you from your body. Many of them can't be seen by other people, are often difficult to describe, and are usually unpredictable. Also, even though you may have symptoms which can be called the same name as those experienced by others, your experience of them is completely personal. The times when they occur, the level of intensity, the effect on you—these are entirely individual. In addition, common symptoms—fatigue, stress, shortness of breath, pain, itching, anger, depression, and sleep problems—can interact with each other in a manner particular to your situation. This interaction can, in turn, worsen existing symptoms and may lead to new ones. It can be a real tangle.

However, there are practical ways of approaching the management of your symptoms, using action-planning based on information gathered by you about your own situation. The next chapter, chapter 5, looks at "cognitive" techniques, which are mental tools—ways you can use your mind to help deal with your symptoms, in addition to the practical points in this chapter.

Dealing with Common Symptoms

You are the expert on your own symptoms, common or not. That means you are in a position to apply problem-solving procedures to the self-management of your symptoms; in other words, you can develop action plans in this area of your life—look at chapter 2 to remind yourself of the stages. Your goal is to reduce or remove the bother or the discomfort of a particular symptom, so that your life gets easier. Before you can manage a symptom, you need to identify what it is, so a first step is to track back to the cause—or causes—and at that point you will be in a much better position to form an action plan and do something. While this may sound like a simple and obvious process, it is not always easy because in a chronic condition, each symptom may have many causes, the symptoms themselves may be inter-related and many of them get in the way of clear, positive thinking.

One way to untangle the threads is to keep a daily diary or journal. This can be as simple as writing your symptoms and what you are doing on a calendar, or in a notebook which you may use for other self-management records, to do with diet and exercise, for example. Writing things down helps to clarify your thoughts, and it also helps you remember. After a week or two, you will probably see a pattern. For example, you go out to dinner on Saturday evening and wake up in the night with stomach ache. You realise that when you go out you overeat. Next time you can adjust what you order. Every time you go dancing your feet hurt, but this does not happen when you walk. Maybe the different shoes you wear cause the pain. Seeing patterns is for many the first step towards symptom self-management. See page 33 for an example of a sample calendar journal. Keeping a journal like this can be really helpful in finding patterns. Having found these patterns, some people keep going with writing down their symptoms and continue to find this helpful. Others find that continuing to write down symptoms makes them notice the symptoms even more, so they appear worse. You might want to find out what works best for you.

Looking at this person's sample calendar, we can see the following patterns:

- Something happens when the person is baby-sitting that causes pain—maybe it is lifting, chasing after small children, or leaning over to change diapers.
- When this person has pain she tends to be tired the next day.
- Water exercise makes her feel better, although she may be a little stiff the next day.
- Eating dinner out seems to result in poor sleep and being tired the next day. Maybe she eats too much, or maybe this is the only time she drinks alcohol. Even a little alcohol at night can interfere with good-quality sleep.

SAMPLE CALENDAR JOURNAL

Mon	Tue	Wed	Thur	Fri	Sat	Sun
Grocery shop	Baby-sit grand kids Pain PM	Tired	Water exercise Feel great	Little stiff Clean house	Dinner out Poor sleep	Tired

Mon	Tue	Wed	Thur	Fri	Sat	Sun
Grocery shop	Baby-sit grandkids	Tired	Water exercise	Clean house	Feel Great	Feel Great Dinner Out Poor sleep

So, as you read through this chapter, you may find that many symptoms have the same causes. Also, one symptom may actually cause other symptoms. When you understand better the possible causes of your symptoms, it may be easier for you to work out how to manage them. You may also find ways to prevent some of them from coming back.

Now, here are some of the more common symptoms experienced by people with different chronic conditions—fatigue, stress, shortness of breath, pain, itching, anger, depression and sleep problems.

Fatigue

Having a chronic illness can drain your energy. Fatigue is a real problem and not "all in the mind". It can stop you doing things you really want to do. Unfortunately, other people sometimes do not understand how fatigue can suddenly hit you. They may think you are not interested or that you want to be alone and are just making an excuse.

To manage your fatigue, it may help you to be aware that there can be many reasons for it. These may include the disease itself, not being active, poor diet, weight problems, emotions, not enough sleep and, sometimes, medication. Once again, a daily record or journal of symptoms may be a valuable self-management tool. You can begin to sort out whether some of these possible reasons apply to you.

- **The disease itself.** To do anything, you need energy. When you have a chronic illness, your body uses up energy to heal itself. This means you may have less energy left for everyday activities.
- **Not being active**. When you don't use muscles, they become wasted and don't work well. The heart is made of muscular tissue and as such, it can also become less efficient. This means the heart will be less good at pumping blood, which carries necessary nutrients and oxygen around the body. When muscles do not get food and oxygen, they cannot work properly. They get tired more easily than muscles that are in good condition.
- **Poor diet.** Food is our basic source of energy. If you eat too much junk food or don't eat the right amount of food, you can get fatigued more easily. If your fatigue is caused by not eating well, then the solution is to eat better-quality foods in the proper quantities. If you can't eat much and are losing weight, the quality of food you eat is very important. Chapter 12 discusses, in greater detail, some of the problems associated with eating, as well as tips for improving your eating habits.
- **Weight problems.** Carrying too much weight around can lead to fatigue, because it causes an increase in the amount of energy you need to do anything else. Being underweight can also lead to fatigue. People often say they can't exercise because they feel fatigued. Believing this creates a vicious circle. People are fatigued because of lack of exercise, and yet they don't exercise because of the fatigue. Believe it or not, if this is your problem, then motivating yourself to do a little exercise the next time you feel tired (unless it's bedtime anyway!) might be the answer. You don't have to run a marathon. The important thing is to get outdoors and take a short walk. If this is not possible, then walk around your house. See chapter 6 for more information on getting started on an exercise programme.

- **Emotions.** Feeling under stress, anxious, fearful or depressed can also use up energy. There is a section on how to deal with depression a little later in this chapter. If you feel that your fatigue may be related to stress, then read the next section for some tips on managing stress.

- **Not enough sleep.** Most people are aware of the connection between being stressed and feeling tired, but fewer are aware that fatigue is also a symptom of depression. If this is the case, rest will probably not help. In fact, it may make you feel worse. There is a section on how to deal with depression a little later in this chapter.

- **Medications.** Some medicines can cause fatigue. If you think your fatigue is medication-related, talk to your doctor. Sometimes your medication or the dose can be changed.

There are sections on stress, sleep, depression and medication later in this chapter. Exercise and healthy eating have chapters of their own.

So, if fatigue is a problem, your first job, as a self-manager who wants to minimise the symptom and its effect on your life, is to determine the cause. In your journal, you may find you are answering the following questions. Are you eating healthy foods? Are you exercising? Are you getting enough good-quality sleep? If you answer "no" to any of these questions, you may be well on your way to determining one or more of the reasons, other than your illness, for your fatigue. Once you've established a possible cause of your fatigue, you can start work on an action-plan as outlined in chapter 2. That means, you will think about your symptom afresh, identify it exactly, think what you might do about it, and choose something to try, to improve the situation.

Stress

Stress is a common problem for everybody. But what is stress? In the 1950s, physiologist Hans Selye described stress as "the nonspecific response of the body to any demand made upon it." The body adapts to demands, whether pleasant or unpleasant. For example, sitting in the sun on a warm spring day, you may relax. Your blood pressure and pulse will go down. Being caught in a cold, driving rain will cause your body to speed up. Your blood pressure and pulse will go up. In short, you are stressed.

Your body is used to working at a certain level. When you have to do something extra, your body prepares for physical action and makes sure oxygen and energy are sent to your muscles. This causes your breathing to speed up, your heart rate to increase. Your blood pressure rises, your digestion slows, your neck and shoulder muscles tense, your mouth becomes dry and you may begin sweating.

Why does this happen? To make a movement, your muscles need to be supplied with oxygen and energy. Your rate of breathing increases in an effort to inhale as much oxygen as possible and to get rid of as much carbon dioxide as possible. Your heart rate increases to deliver the oxygen and nutrients via the blood supply to the muscles. Furthermore, physiological processes that are not immediately necessary, such as the digestion of food and the body's natural immune responses, are slowed down. Strangely enough, these things happen even when you do not need more oxygen, such as when you are afraid or anxious.

How long will these responses last? In general, only until the event passes. Then your body returns to normal. Sometimes, though, your body does not return to its former comfortable level. If stress is present for any length of time, your body begins adapting to that. This adaptation can contribute to other problems, such as hypertension, shortness of breath, or muscle and joint pain.

Knowing that these are the body's response to stress may help you recognise and then manage related symptoms.

Common Types of Stressors

It also helps to recognise some commonly stressful situations. Stressors are the "something extra" that your body has to cope with. Stressors are activities, incidents, feelings or anything that causes stress.

A few examples of stressors are the following:

- **Physical stressors.** These increase your body's demand for energy. A physical stressor can be something pleasant like picking up your grandchild for the first time, or it could be a big shopping trip demanding a lot of energy. The physical symptoms of your illness can be stressors. If your body is not prepared to deal with the demand for energy, you may get sore muscles or even a worsening of disease symptoms.

- **Chemical stressors.** Cigarettes, coffee, alcohol or drugs can act as chemical stressors.
- **Mental and emotional stressors.** These can range from pleasant to uncomfortable feelings. Joyful experiences such as family weddings lead to the same stress response in your body as feeling frustrated or down because of your illness. It may seem odd but it is simply the way the stress is perceived by your brain and reacted to by your body.
- **Environmental stressors.** These can also include both good and bad things like a sunny day, uneven pavements that make it difficult to walk, loud noises, or smoky rooms.
- **Good stressors.** Some types of stress can be good, such as a job promotion, a wedding, a vacation, a new friendship, or a new baby. These stressors make you feel happy, but still cause the physiological changes in your body that were discussed above. Exercise is another example of a good stress that puts demands on your body. Your heart works harder to get blood to the muscles, your lungs work harder and you breathe more quickly to keep up with your muscles' need for oxygen. Your muscles are working hard to keep up with signals from your brain telling them to keep moving. As you keep up your exercise programme for several weeks, you begin to see changes. What seemed nearly impossible at the start is now much easier. Your body has adapted to the stress. There is less strain on your heart, lungs and muscles which are more efficient. You have become more fit.

What all these stressors have in common is that they increase your body's need for energy.

Recognising When You Feel Stressed

Stress is helpful as long as you do not go past your 'breaking point'. Some days you can tolerate more stress than others. Other days, though, if you are not aware of stress, you can go beyond breaking point, and feel as if your whole life is out of control. In order to monitor your stress level, you could look out for some of these signs:

- Biting your nails, pulling your hair, other repetitive habits;
- Grinding your teeth, clenching your jaw;
- Tensing your head, neck or shoulders;
- Feeling anxious, nervous, helpless or irritable;
- Having many accidents or forgetting things you don't normally forget.

Dealing with Stress

Problem Solving

Notice that stress is building up. You can see stressful situations outside you and you can feel a stressed response inside you. The first step is start listening to and recognising your own body's signals that stress is building up internally. The list of possible signs above may help you. Stress can get in the way of really good problem solving, so learning to stand outside the situation and think objectively is a first step, and noticing our own early stress responses can save creating further symptom tangles.

You may know already of some external situations you always find stressful, such as going on a long journey or preparing a meal. Using problem-solving procedures, track back to what it is about the situation that you find stressful. Is it that you hate to be late? Do you worry about parking? Does cooking demand too much energy? Then begin to look for options open to you to reduce the stress. You could leave earlier. You could use public transport. For a meal in the evening, you could do part of the preparation in the morning, part in the afternoon. You could have a fifteen-minute nap in the afternoon. List some options, choose one and try it next time you are in this kind of situation. Don't forget to evaluate the results, because if the first option doesn't work, you are in a position to try the next with a new action plan.

In a stressful situation, the temptation can be to smoke a cigarette, drink a glass of wine or a cup of coffee. This seems to help, but the effect is only temporary. What's more, nicotine, alcohol and caffeine actually cause their own sets of uncomfortable and stressful symptoms. Cutting them out, or at least cutting them down, can leave you feeling calmer. Being calmer lets you think more effectively about ways to solve the problems.

There are other ways to deal with stress. These are techniques where you use your mind. They include self-talk, progressive muscle relaxation, guided imagery, and visualisation—have a look at chapter 5. Exercising— chapters 6, 7 and 8—and eating healthily—chapter 12—contribute to coping better with stress.

Sometimes stress is so overwhelming that a good self-manager will realise they could do with help. This is the time to approach your consultants - your doctor, a counsellor, social worker, psychologist or psychiatrist. If you can't solve a problem yourself, it is only common sense, and excellent self-management, to see someone who can.

Once you have recognised you are under stress, there are many options open to you. Following up one option to problem-solve in one area of your life can be the step that breaks the cycle of stress from elsewhere.

Shortness of Breath

Chronic illness can lead to changes in the body which cause breathlessness. The situations in which you notice it may differ from one person to another. For one, walking uphill may cause distress, while another may have trouble in a smoky room. Knowing some of the possible bodily reasons for feeling breathless might help you begin to solve your own problem. These include:

- Air sacs in the lungs that are not working well, preventing the lungs getting oxygen into the blood and carbon dioxide out of the blood;
- Narrowing of the airways to the air sacs and over-secretion of mucus, which reduces air flow to the lungs;
- The heart not pumping blood efficiently, so blood doesn't get through the lungs as well as it might. This leads to the lungs being less stretchy and more difficult to fill with air, leading to breathlessness.;
- Being overweight which increases the amount of energy and oxygen the body needs so that the heart has to work harder;
- Deconditioning of the muscles which empty and fill the lungs, which can make breathing feel harder work, because the process is less efficient.

Managing Shortness of Breath

When you feel short of breath, don't stop what you are doing or hurry to finish, but slow down and work out how you feel. Often, shortness of breath is frightening, and the fear itself can cause two additional problems. First, the hormones that fear can release may cause more shortness of breath. Second, fear may cause you to stop your activity and thus never build up the endurance necessary to help your breathing. The basic rule is to take things slowly and in steps. Develop goals and an action plan.

- **Increase your activity level gradually, generally not by more than 25% each week.** If you are now able to garden comfortably for twenty minutes, next week increase it by a maximum of five minutes. Once you can garden comfortably for twenty-five minutes, you can again add a few more.
- **Don't smoke, and avoid smokers.** This may sometimes be difficult, because smoking friends may not realise how difficult they are making your life. Your job is to tell them. Explain that their smoke is causing breathing problems for you and that you would appreciate it if they would not smoke when you are around. Also, make your house and especially your car "No Smoking" zones. Ask people to smoke outside.
- **Use your medication and oxygen as prescribed by your doctor.** We are constantly being bombarded by messages that drugs are bad and not to be used. In some cases, this is correct. However, when you have a chronic condition, drugs can be, and often are, life savers. Don't try to skimp, cut down, or go without. More is not better, so don't take more than the prescribed amount of medicine. Drugs, taken as prescribed, can make all the difference. This may mean using medication even when you are not having symptoms. It also means resisting the temptation to take an extra dose if the prescribed amount does not seem to be working. If you have questions about your medicines or feel they are not working for you, talk to your doctor before you either stop taking the medication or increase the dose. Develop a medication action plan with your doctor. Preventing problems before they start is much better than having to manage the problems. Chapter 13 discusses some issues around managing your medicines.

- **Drink plenty of fluids if mucus and secretions are a problem.** —Unless your doctor has advised you to restrict your fluid intake. Drinking enough will help thin the mucus and, therefore, make it easier to cough up. The use of a humidifier may also be helpful because it keeps the air around you moist.

Develop your breathing control with diaphragmatic breathing. Diaphragmatic breathing is also called breathing control and belly breathing. As mentioned earlier, one of the problems that can cause shortness of breath is deconditioning of the diaphragm and breathing muscles. When this deconditioning occurs, the lungs can't expand and contract to their fullest extent. That is, they do not fill well, nor do they get rid of old air. Diaphragmatic breathing strengthens the breathing muscles. With more efficient breathing muscles, you have to put less energy into your breathing. It is worth putting in some practice to master the technique.

Here are some steps to help you learn how to control your breathing:

1. Lie on your back with pillows under your head and knees. Place one hand on your stomach, below your breastbone or sternum, and the other hand on your upper chest. Breathe in slowly through your nose, allowing your stomach to expand outward. Imagine that your lungs are getting filled with fresh air. The hand on your stomach should move upward, and the hand on your chest should not move or only move slightly. Breathe out slowly, through pursed lips. At the same time, use your hand to gently push inward and upward on your abdomen. Practise this technique for ten to fifteen minutes, three or four times a day, until it becomes automatic. If you begin to feel a bit dizzy, rest.

2. When you are comfortable doing this, you can place a light weight on your abdomen. This will help to strengthen the muscles you use to breathe in. Start with a weight of about one pound (500 grams) like a book or a bag of rice or beans. Over the weeks, increase the weight as your muscle strength improves.

3. You can also practise diaphragmatic breathing while sitting in a chair. Relax your shoulders, arms, hands, and chest. Do not

Positions That Will Help If You Are Breathless or Short of Breath

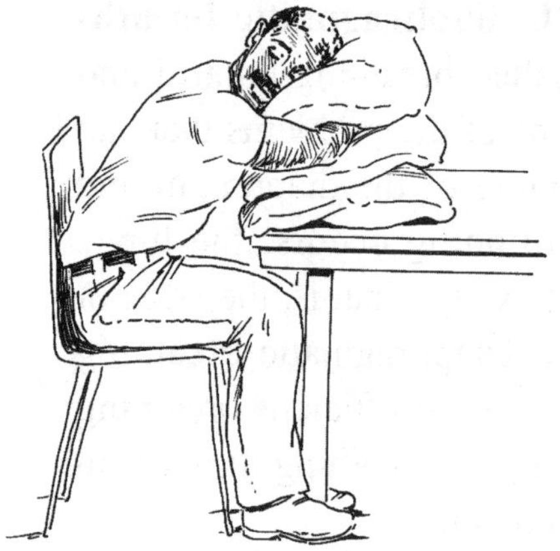

Forward lean sitting

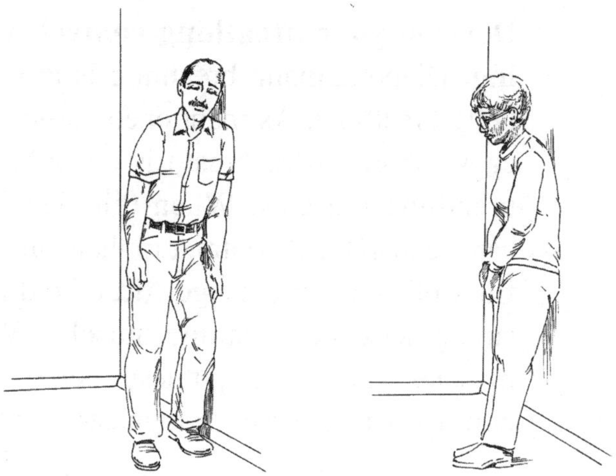

Standing

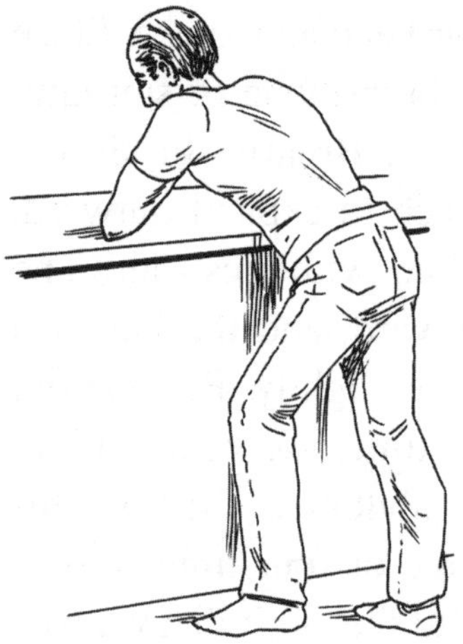

Forward lean standing

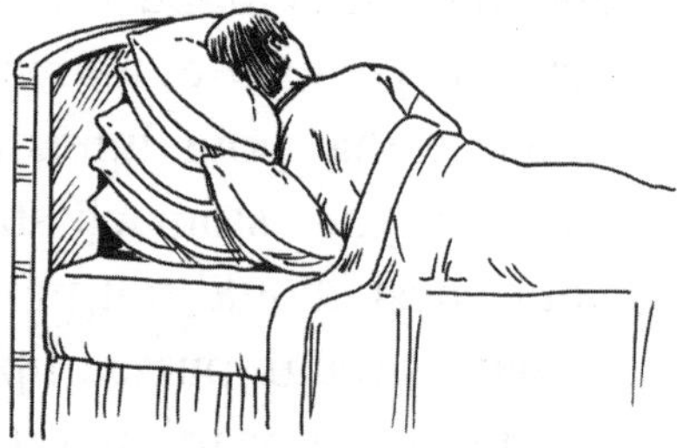

Lying

grip the arms of the chair or your knees. Put one hand on your abdomen and the other on your chest. Breathe in through your nose, filling the area around your waist with air. Your chest hand should remain still and the hand on your abdomen should move. Breathe out without force or effort.

4. Once you are comfortable with this technique, you can practise it at almost any time, lying down, sitting, standing, or walking. Diaphragmatic breathing can help strengthen and improve the coordination and efficiency of the breathing muscles, as well as decrease the amount of energy you need to breathe. You can also use it alongside any of the relaxation techniques that use the power of your mind to manage your symptoms, as described in chapter 5.

Once you are in charge of how you breathe while you are doing other activities, you will be better able to manage your shortness of breath.

- **Develop pursed-lip breathing.** A second technique, pursed-lip breathing, usually happens naturally for people who have problems emptying their lungs. It can also be used if you are short of breath or breathless. Purse your lips as if blowing across a flute or into a whistle. Use diaphragmatic breathing (breathing control). Breathe out through pursed lips without any force. Remember to relax the upper chest, shoulders, arms, and hands while breathing out. Check for tension. Breathing out should take longer than breathing in.

  Again, once you can remember to use this technique while you are doing something else, you are better equipped to manage breathlessness.

- **Clear narrowed airways.** If your sense of being short of breath is caused by over-secretion of mucus or phlegm, which is difficult to clear, you could try huffing, and controlled coughing, two techniques that may be helpful for clearing smaller and larger airways.

Huffing

This technique combines one or two forced huffs with diaphragmatic breathing–breathing control. It is useful for removing secretions from the small airways.

Take in a breath as you would do for diaphragmatic breathing. Hold your breath for a moment. Huff—keep your mouth open while squeezing your chest and abdominal muscles to force out the air, a bit like panting. If possible, do another huff before taking in another breath. Take two or three diaphragmatic breaths. Huff once or twice.

Controlled Coughing

This helps to remove secretions—the phlegm—from larger airways. Take in a full, slow breath—a diaphragmatic breath. Keep shoulders and hand relaxed. Hold the breath for a moment. Cough, that is, tighten the abdominal muscles and force the air out. Note: If you have a bout of uncontrolled coughing, this may help: Avoid very dry air or steam. Swallow as soon as the bout starts. Sip water. Suck lozenges or a hard sweet. Try diaphragmatic breathing, being sure to breathe in through your nose.

Pain and Physical Discomfort

Pain or physical discomfort is a problem shared by many people with chronic illness. In fact, for many people, this is their number one concern. As with most symptoms of chronic illness, pain or discomfort can have many causes.

The five most common causes are:

- **The disease itself.** Pain can be due to inflammation, damage in or around joints and tissues, lack of proper blood supply to the heart, damage to the nervous system or trapped nerves, amongst other causes.
- **Tense muscles.** When something hurts, the muscles in that area become tense. This is your body's natural reaction to pain, to try to protect the area that is damaged. When muscles are tensed for a long time, lactic acid builds up in the muscles and this can also cause soreness or pain.
- **Muscle deconditioning.** With a chronic condition, it is common to become less active, leading to a weakening of the muscles, or muscle deconditioning. When a muscle is weak, it tends to complain any time it is used. Even the slightest activity can sometimes lead to pain and stiffness.

- **Lack of sleep, or poor quality sleep.** Pain can stop you either getting to sleep or having a good sleep. This, in turn, can make pain worse and leave you less able to cope with it.
- **Emotions and stress.** Anxiety, depression, anger, fear and frustration are all normal responses to living with a chronic condition, and they can affect the way you feel pain. eing stressed, angry, afraid or depressed, can make everything, including the pain and discomfort worse, both by making muscles more tense and painful and by making the nerves that carry pain signals more sensitive.
- **Medication.** The medicine you are taking can sometimes cause pain and discomfort. If you suspect this, talk to your doctor.

Managing Pain

Because pain comes from many sources, the methods we use to manage or reduce pain must take into account its cause in our own condition.

Many people who have persistent pain get into the habit of allowing their pain to decide what and how much they do. In itself, this is sensible, of course, when pain is the body's suggestion to the mind that it needs to stop. However, in terms of action-planning to manage pain, it may lead to using the onset or worsening of pain as the planned stopping point for an activity. You may as a result always, more or less consciously, link activities with pain – because you always go on until it hurts too much. You may have internalised the notion "I had to stop because it was painful" or even "I can't ever do that because it always hurts". This can feed into frustration, anger and resentment about your condition, all complicating the symptom cycle.

Ask yourself these questions when you are considering how to plan an approach to the symptom of pain. First, do you do more on good days and less on bad days? Second, do you normally do more than you have to – that is, do you habitually over-achieve? Third, do you feel you have to finish something just because you've started it? Fourth, do you have a problem saying no when people ask you to do things? If you answer yes to any or all of these, you may be into a cycle of over and under-achievement which is set up and driven by the pain which you are setting out to manage. You work hard and over-achieve when you feel all right, you keep going till you feel bad, and then you are forced to do nothing in order to recuperate, under-achieving for a day or two. Of course, by this stage, you may be tempted to work too hard to catch up with whatever jobs have been waiting for you and the cycle starts again. The answer is to pace yourself.

Pacing is spacing your activities out through the day. Pacing is getting on with something, but taking a break before you need to. Pacing is prioritising your goals and working towards them in manageable stages.

Action-planning is a good way to break into the cycle and to put pacing yourself at the centre of whatever you do. You have carried out stages 1 – 4 towards your goal of, say, clearing and replanting a flowerbed in the garden. You reach action-plan stage 5 where you check on progress. You find you haven't got as far as you wanted because pain has prevented you from completing the clearing. At stage 6, you plan changes to deal with this unforeseen problem. Analysing the problem reveals to you that you worked for a substantial period without too much bother – the pain only came on after an hour. So the revised action plan now includes precise timing. You plan to stop after twenty minutes, even if there is no pain, and to wait till next day to start again. You carry out the new plan strictly, using a clock or a timer and stopping when you planned to. As you get stronger, or more flexible, or whatever improvement you gain from working in the garden, you can review the plan again and extend your working time. You have managed your life in such a way that this aspect of it is no longer dominated by the symptom of pain—you have taken control of it yourself.

Some kinds of pain can be relieved by medicine, for example, those that open blood vessels and bronchial tubes and those that reduce inflammation.

Two of the best ways to deal with pain are the use of exercise—chapters 6, 7 and 8 and symptom management techniques that use your mind, such as relaxation and visualisation—chapter 5. In addition, there are several other methods that are sometimes useful for pain in particular spots. These include the use of heat, cold, and massage. These three applications work by stimulating the skin and other tissues surrounding the painful area, which in turn increases the blood flow to these areas.

Stimulation with heat can be done by applying a heating pad or by taking a warm bath or shower, with the water flow directed at the painful area. You can make a heating "pad" by placing rice or dry beans in a sock, knotting the top of the sock, and placing it in a microwave oven for a few minutes. Before use, be sure to test the heat so as not to burn yourself. Do not use popcorn. Leave it in place for fifteen to twenty minutes, no longer.

Cold applications suit some people better, for soothing pain, especially if there is inflammation. You can use a bag of frozen peas or corn which makes a cheap, reusable cold pack. Put a cloth between your skin and the cold. (Don't eat them once they're thawed and re-frozen!) As with a hot pack, leave it in place for no more than twenty minutes.

Massage is one of the oldest forms of pain management. Hippocrates (c. 460–380 B.C.) said, "Physicians must be experienced in many things, but assuredly also in the rubbing that can bind a joint that is loose and loosen a joint that is too hard." Self-massage is a simple procedure, for the bits of you that you can reach, that can be performed with little practice or preparation. It stimulates the skin, the underlying tissues and the muscles. There are plenty of good creams to massage into your skin.

However, don't use self-massage for a "hot joint"—one that is red, swollen, and hot to the touch—or an infected area, nor if you are suffering from phlebitis, thrombophlebitis, or skin eruptions.

Once again, if self-management tools can't do all you want, the next step is to ask for help. If pain continues to have a major influence on your life, it is not a sign of failure to ask for a referral to a pain management clinic. It is sensible self-management.

Itching

Itching is a difficult symptom to understand and is even harder to define. Basically, itching is any sensation that causes an urge to scratch. It can have many different causes. Some of these we understand, such as the itching caused by the release of histamines that irritate nerve endings. This happens when you get an insect bite or come in contact with a substance such as stinging nettles. People with liver diseases may also experience itching that is caused by bile products deposited in the skin, when the liver is damaged and can't function properly. Kidney disease may lead to severe itching but we don't know why. There are other conditions, such as the skin condition psoriasis, where the cause of the itching is not easily explained. We do know that other factors such as warmth, wool clothing, and stress can make itching worse.

Managing and Relieving Itching

Use Moisture

Dry skin tends to be itchy so moisturise your skin with cream several times a day. When you choose a moisturiser, be careful to check what the ingredients are. If alcohol or any other ingredient that ends in "ol", which is usually some variant of alcohol, appears on the list, don't use it, because these tend actually to dry the skin. In general, the greasier the product, the better it works as a moisturiser.

Creams are better moisturisers than lotions, and products such as Vaseline, olive or vegetable oils are also very effective.

When taking a bath or a shower, use warm water and soak for between ten and twenty minutes. You also may want to add bath oil or bicarbonate of soda—or a mixture of two teaspoons of olive oil in a large glass of milk, added to the bath water, which has a good moisturising effect. Pat yourself dry immediately and apply your cream.

If something in contact with your skin has set off an itchy allergic reaction, wash off the substance, apply a cold compress and take an antihistamine medicine, such as diphenhydramine (Benadryl).

Use a humidifier at home and at work during the winter, because indoor heating tends to dry the air, and your skin.

Wear Natural Fibres Next to Your Skin

The type of clothing you wear can make your itching worse, so choose comfortable materials. Polyester, nylon and acrylic fabrics can be uncomfortable. Most people find that natural fibres, such as cotton, linen and silk, and also rayon and viscose, allow the skin to "breathe" better. Read the labels.

Use Your Medication

Antihistamines will help if your itching is caused by the release of histamines. You can buy many of these products over the counter (OTC). Ask your doctor or pharmacist for advice, and do not use a cream for a long time without talking to your doctor. If your itching carries on even with OTC products, you may want to talk to your doctor about trying stronger prescription version of these medications.

Reduce Stress

Anything that you can do to reduce the stress in your life will also help reduce itching. We have already discussed some of the ways to deal with stress earlier in this chapter, and there are some other techniques in chapter 5.

Don't Scratch

It is a natural reaction to scratch what itches, but many people find it does not help, especially for chronic itching. The more you scratch, the more you itch. It is an understatement to say that it is hard to resist scratching, but you might try rubbing, pressing or patting the skin instead. Again, this may be a time to talk to one of your consultants, perhaps a professional skin specialist. Your doctor may be able to suggest other ways of controlling itching and to offer prescription medicines to help with specific types of itching.

Anger

Anger is one of the most common responses to chronic illness. "Why me?" The uncertainty and unpredictability of living with a chronic disease threatens what you have worked all your life to achieve – independence and control. The loss of control over one's body and loss of independence in life can create feelings of frustration, helplessness and hopelessness, all of which fuel the anger. You may sometimes have found yourself wondering what you did to deserve this. All these are very common, even normal anger responses to chronic disease.

You may be angry with yourself, family, friends, health care providers, God, or the world in general – all for a variety of reasons. For example, you may be angry with yourself for not taking better care of yourself when you were younger. You may be angry with your family and friends because they don't do things the way you would like them done. Or you might be angry with your doctor because they can't solve your problems. Sometimes your anger might be misplaced, such as when you find yourself shouting at the cat. Misplaced anger is quite common, especially if you are not even aware that you are angry, let alone why.

Sometimes anger is not just a response to having a chronic illness, but is actually a result of the disease process. For example, if someone has suffered a stroke that has affected a certain part of the brain, that person's ability to express or suppress emotions may be affected. So some people who have strokes may appear to cry inappropriately or have outbursts of temper.

You can learn how to manage anger, the same as any other symptom. Recognising and then acknowledging that you are angry and identifying why, or with whom, are important steps in learning how to manage it effectively. Anger needs to be expressed – the task is to find ways of doing so constructively. If it isn't expressed, it can become unhealthy. It can build up until it becomes explosive and offends others, or is turned inwards, intensifying the experience of other disease symptoms like depression.

There are several things you can do to help manage your anger.

- **Communicate it in words.** You can do it without blaming or offending others. Use "I", rather than "You" messages, to express your feelings. Look at Chapter 9 Communicating for discussion of "I" messages. However, something that needs remembering is that, even when you have learnt how to express your anger verbally, you may well still have to allow for the fact that other people might not be able to help you. Many of us are not very good at handling other people's anger, even if it is justified and even if we want to help. Try to keep the lines of communication open.

- **Find places outside your home to express anger.** You might increase your self-management skills by finding other places to express and speak about your anger, such as counselling or a support group, where you can find healthy release for your angry feelings in words in a supportive situation.

- **Modify your expectations.** We all do this as a perfectly normal process throughout our lives. As a child, we think we can become anything—a fireman, a ballet dancer, a doctor—but as we grow and learn, we change our expectations in accordance with what we know of our capabilities, talents and interests. Based on continual re-evaluation, we keep on modifying our plans. You can consciously use the same process to deal with the effects of chronic illness on your life. It may be unrealistic to expect that you will get completely better, but it is perfectly realistic to expect that you can still do many pleasurable things. You have the ability to affect the progress of your illness, by slowing its decline or preventing it from becoming worse. Changing your expectations can help you to change the way you look at things. Instead of dwelling on the 10% of things you can't do any more, you can choose to focus on the 90% of things you can do. You may well be able to find new activities or hobbies to replace lost ones.

- **Take up new activities.** Anger can often be caused by pent up energy that is not being released. Having anger inside means that you have energy going to waste; you can express your anger through exercise, writing, music or painting. Some people find these very therapeutic, because once again, anger can be released in a healthy way. Once it has been noticed, expressed and listened to, by you, you can move on.

- **Develop a positive attitude.** Use positive "self-talk" help change your perspective instead of using energy being angry. There is more about this in the next chapter.

Anger is not in itself a bad thing. It is energy for change. It is a normal response to having a chronic condition. Part of learning to live a healthy life with your condition is to pay attention to your anger, and then to manage it to help you move along and change your life for the better.

Depression

"Depression" can be a frightening word. Some people prefer to say they are "sad" or "feeling down" or "a bit low". Whatever you call it, some feeling like this is a very common, normal reaction to chronic illness. If your disease is a significant problem in your life, you almost certainly have or have had some experience of depression.

We discussed some of the common factors in the situation of people with chronic disease when we looked at why you have probably felt angry, in the section above. Depression can also result from such situations and, being inter-related with other symptoms, can develop in a downward spiral. Just as there are many degrees of pain, there are different degrees of depression. It can be difficult to recognise when you are becoming depressed, but the art of self-management is to spot the signs, work out what you can do about them, and catch yourself before you fall into a deeper state.

People experience feelings about a chronic condition which, of course, are entirely personal, but which they may well have in common with others. Many of these feelings can use up energy and, unless they are worked through, can lead to depression.

- **Fear, anxiety and worry about your future.** Whether these feelings are to do with the disease process, treatment, your family or finances, working with them early on will make them less likely to lead to depression. By dealing with any specific problem that is making you anxious, you and others involved in any of your anxieties will spend less time worrying and more enjoying life. Chapter 15 deals with certain decisions we all have to make at some time in our lives. If the issues are clarified in your own mind and with your family, you will find you are less uncertain about the future.

- **Frustration, which can have any number of causes.** You may find yourself thinking, "I can't just do what I want," "I feel so helpless," "I used to be able to do this myself," or "Why doesn't anyone understand me?" Thoughts like these can increase frustration and leave you feeling more alone and isolated which, in turn, can feed depression.

- **Feeling you have lost control of your life.** This may come from having to rely on medication to ease symptoms, having to depend on others to help you perform daily activities such as bathing, dressing or preparing meals or having to visit outpatients or the doctor on a regular basis. This feeling of losing control can make you lose faith in yourself and your abilities, which can be depressing.

Although they can be described as if they are separate, these feelings are often experienced in combination, making it difficult to reach the root cause of the depression. Also, the need to appear positive to family and friends may lead some people to be outwardly cheerful and to refuse offers of help. That may make it harder to be honest inside, to admit to ourselves that we are actually depressed. But that has to be done as a first step to confronting depression. As with anger, it can be difficult to recognise exactly what you are feeling. It is, however, perfectly possible to learn to recognise it, accept it and manage it. Look at chapter 15 as well.

The first step is to spot the signs of depression.

Recognising Depression

The following are common signs of depression that you can learn to recognise

- A general feeling of unhappiness that won't go away
- A loss of interest in life, not able to enjoy anything, avoiding people, not wanting to answer the phone or the doorbell
- Loss of interest in personal care and grooming
- Difficulty in making simple decisions, inability to concentrate
- Loss of energy, feeling very tired all the time
- Feeling restless and twitchy
- Changed eating habits, from loss of interest in food to unusually erratic or excessive eating
- Difficulty sleeping, or sleeping too much
- Loss of interest in being held or in sex. Sometimes this can be due to side-effects of medication. Talk this over with your doctor
- Loss of self-confidence, low self-image, feeling useless

- Suicidal thoughts. If your unhappiness has caused you to think about killing yourself, tell someone and get help from close friends, a social worker, a member of your church, a psychologist or a doctor. Such feelings pass and you will feel better, so get help
- Frequent accidents. Watch for a pattern of increased carelessness, accidents while walking or driving, dropping things – though take account of the physical problems which might be caused by your condition, such as unsteady balance or slowed reaction times
- Irritability, getting into frequent arguments over minor matters that did not bother you before.

The behaviour of a person who is depressed and trying to cover it up, may give some clues to those around them. Over-cheerfulness alongside continual refusal of offers of help, even when obviously needed, may be recognised by a wise observer. If behaviour tends to be excessive in one direction or another from what would be considered normal for that person, this may often be a sign of unrecognised depression. The paradox of depression-related behaviour is that the more obviously and frequently it occurs, the more likely it is that it will alienate those who most want to help, and are most capable of providing the comfort and support the depressed person needs. Most of our friends and family want to help us feel better, but often they don't really know what to do to help. As their efforts to comfort and reassure us are frustrated, they may at some point throw up their hands and stop trying. Then the depressed person is confirmed in their belief that no-one cares, increasing their depression by the sense of loss and loneliness.

You may be familiar with some of these signs of depression. They are very common amongst people with chronic illness. Whether you've experienced them in the past or now, you share the experience with many others. Also along with many others, you can get to grips with aspects of your situation and your feelings, to manage your depression. If you are depressed, you may not feel like making the effort. However, you can decide to act in spite of that. You can force yourself into the first step towards breaking out of it. Ask for help with that step – find someone to talk to. If you have people living with you, you might talk to them. If you live on your own – and having a chronic illness while living alone can be very depressing - you will need to look outside for someone you can talk to. Nobody can tell you how you should or should not feel, but most people probably generally agree that being depressed is not pleasant. It is, happily, true that we don't need to put up with it, and active self-management can move us on.

Managing Depression

- **If you feel like hurting yourself or someone else, ring your doctor, a religious leader, a care professional, local community centre, local support agency or national organisations like the Samaritans or NHS Direct (0845 4647).** Don't wait. Very often, just talking to someone who understands why you need to talk will be enough to help you through this mood. Do it right now.

- **Don't take tranquillisers or narcotic painkillers such as morphine, oxycodone or fentanyl, or medication to help you sleep.** These drugs intensify depression, and the sooner you can stop taking them, the better. Your depression may be a drug side-effect. If you are not sure what you are taking or uncertain if what you're experiencing could be a side-effect, check with your doctor or your pharmacist. Don't stop taking a prescription drug without checking with the person who prescribed it. There may be important reasons for carrying on with it, perhaps withdrawal reactions you need to know about. Talk to your doctor.

- **Don't drink alcohol.** Alcohol is a "downer"—it can cheer you up briefly but the longer effect is depressing. Unless you keep your brain clear of the negative effects of alcohol, you will find it almost impossible to avoid depression. For most people, one or two drinks in the evening is not a problem, but if your mind is not free of alcohol during most of the day, you are having trouble with this drug. Talk this over with your doctor, who will have heard many people say the same things, or call Alcoholics Anonymous.

- **Continue your daily activities.** Get washed and dressed every day, make your bed, get out of the house, go shopping, walk your dog. Plan and cook meals regularly. Decide to do these things and force yourself to do them, even if you don't feel like it.

- **Meet your friends.** Ring them up. Visit them. Plan to go to the cinema or other outings. Just do it.

- **Join a group.** Get involved in a church group, a discussion group, an adult education class. If you can't get out, consider a group on the Internet (though make sure the group is moderated and has someone in charge to enforce the rules of the group).

- **Volunteer.** People who help other people are hardly ever depressed.
- **Make plans and carry them out.**
- **Look to the future.** Plant some seeds. Plant a tree. Look forward to your grandchildren's birthdays. Look forward to your own birthday and fix up a treat to celebrate yourself. If you know that one time of the year is especially difficult, such as Christmas, make specific plans for that period. Don't wait to see what happens, expecting it to be a bad period. Take deliberate steps to be prepared.
- **Don't move house without a lot of thought.** Stay for a few weeks in any community you think you might want to live in - don't move house without first staying in the new place to learn what's there for you. Moving can be a sign of withdrawal, and depression can get worse when you are away from friends and acquaintances. Trouble can move with you, whereas the support network you may need to deal with it has to be built again from scratch.
- **Do a day trip.**
- **Go on holiday.** Even a couple of days away with friends or relatives can help.
- **Do a few minutes of physical activity as often as you possibly can.** Natural substances released in the brain have a cheering effect after even moderate exercise.
- **Make a list of rewards for yourself.** Listen to your favourite music, watch a chosen television programme or a DVD. Plan something you can look forward to.
- **Take care of yourself as if you were looking after someone you love.**
- **Use positive self-talk.** This is a cognitive technique which is a very powerful weapon against depression. Look at chapter 5 for more information on "self-talk".
- **Seek professional help.** Often some "talk therapy", with or without medication, can go a long way towards relieving depression.

Seeking professional help and taking medicine are not signs of weakness. They are tools a strong self-manager can choose to use, and making the choice to do so is a sign of strength.

- **Break the cycle.** It is the first step to success in your self-management programme. Depression is not permanent, and you can speed up its departure. Focus on your pride, your friends, your goals, your future and all the positive factors in your surroundings. How you respond to depression can be a self-fulfilling prophecy. When you believe that things can get better, they will.

Sleep Problems

When we are asleep, the body can concentrate on healing itself. Minimal amounts of energy are needed to maintain body functioning while we sleep. When we don't get enough sleep, we can experience a variety of other symptoms, such as fatigue and a lack of concentration. But this does not mean that fatigue and lack of concentration are caused by a lack of sleep. As we discussed in chapter 1, symptoms may be inter-connected and have many causes.

You can apply some practical self-management to the solving of sleep problems and making your night's sleep as refreshing as possible.

Before You Even Get Into Bed

- Get a comfortable bed that allows you to move easily and supports your body well. This usually means a good-quality, firm mattress that supports the spine and keeps the body from rolling only into the middle of the bed. A bed board, made of half-inch to three-quarter-inch (1 or 2 cm) plywood, can be placed between the mattress and the mattress base to increase the firmness.

- Use heat if that helps. Heated water beds or airbeds are helpful for some people because they support weight evenly by conforming to the body's shape—though it's true some people find them very uncomfortable. Having enough warmth from underneath you is important—an electric blanket on low heat or a wool mattress pad is an effective way of keeping properly warm while you are asleep. If you decide on electrically heated bedding be sure to follow the instructions carefully

- Find a comfortable sleeping position. Try using small pillows to help or experiment with larger extra pillows to support your position
- Raise the head of your bed on wooden blocks by about four to six inches to make breathing easier
- Keep your bedroom at a comfortable warm temperature
- Use a vaporiser if the air is dry. Warm and moist air makes breathing easier
- Keep a lamp and telephone beside your bed. Make your bedroom a place in which you feel safe and comfortable
- If you wear glasses or contact lenses during the day, keep a pair of glasses by the bed when you go to sleep. Then if you need to get up in the night, you can see where you are going!

Before Bedtime

- **Avoid eating.** Although you may feel sleepy after eating a big meal, this is not a way to help you fall asleep and get a good night's rest. Digesting food takes energy which is needed during sleep for restoring the body, and that means that your body will not have the energy resources to restore itself. Since going to bed feeling hungry may also keep you awake, try a warm drink- not tea or coffee because of the caffeine—at bedtime

  Avoid alcohol. Contrary to the popular belief that it helps you sleep better, alcohol actually disrupts your sleep cycle. It can lead to shallow and fragmented sleep, as well frequent wakings through the night
- **Avoid caffeine.** Caffeine is a stimulant and it can keep you awake. Caffeine is found in coffee, tea, colas and other soft drinks and chocolate
- **Avoid food with MSG—monosodium glutamate**. Many types of food, especially pre-packaged meals may contain this additive

which can act as a stimulant. Read ingredient labels and ask in restaurants to be sure you don't eat this late in the day

- **Avoid smoking.** Aside from the fact that smoking itself can cause complications and a worsening of your chronic condition, nicotine in cigarettes is a stimulant. And of course, falling asleep with a lit cigarette is a fire hazard
- **Avoid diet pills.** These contain stimulants which may interfere with falling asleep as well as staying asleep

- **Avoid sleeping pills.** While the name "sleeping pills" sounds like the perfect solution to sleep problems, they tend to become less effective over time. Also, if you take them and then stop, it can become even harder to get to sleep
- **Avoid diuretics—water pills.** You may want to take these medicines in the morning so you are not woken by having to get up in the night. Unless your doctor has recommended otherwise, don't reduce the overall amount of fluids you drink, as these are important for your health. However, you might want to limit your fluid intake immediately before you go to bed

Develop a Daily and Nightly Routine By Doing the Following

- **Setting up and keeping to a regular rest and sleep pattern.** Go to bed at the same time every night and get up at the same time every morning. If you need to, take a nap in the afternoon but not after dinner. Stay awake after your evening meal until you are ready for bed
- **Getting your sleep pattern back to normal.** If you are going to bed at 4 a.m. and sleeping until noon, and you want to get back to more usual timing, you can decide to reset your sleep clock. Try going to bed one hour later or earlier each day until you get to the hours you want. This is a way of taking control, and with patience, allowing a new routine to develop
- **Exercising at regular times each day.** Regular exercise can help you sleep well, and it can also help set a regular pattern during your day. It's better not to exercise immediately before bedtime, as it can stimulate you and might keep you awake

- **Getting out in the fresh air and daylight,** even if there's no sun, for fifteen to twenty minutes every day
- **Doing the same things every night before you go to bed.** A 'time-to-get-ready-for-bed' routine such as having a bath and reading a chapter in a book helps your body to wind down and relax
- **Using your bedroom only for sleeping.** If you get into bed and can't fall asleep, get up and go into another room until you begin to feel sleepy again. Your routine is supported by the awareness that, in your bed, you fall asleep easily
- **Using self-management if you wake in the night and have trouble going off again.** Sometimes people go off to sleep easily but wake up and start thinking. Once their mind is active, they find it difficult to drop off again, and it all seems worse when they worry, in addition, that they are not getting enough sleep. Deliberately setting your mind to a task such as counting backwards in threes from 100, or naming a flower for every letter of the alphabet can distract it. Also the relaxation techniques described in the next chapter may help
- **Not worrying about not getting enough sleep.** When your body needs sleep, you will sleep. People tend to need less sleep as they get older, and organising your sleep through the dark hours of the night, when most other people are sleeping, will help you worry less
- **Investigating sleeping too much.** If you find you are able to get to sleep very easily in bed, in the chair and any other time, but are still tired in the day, it may be because you are not breathing properly at night. People who have the most common sleep disorder, called obstructive sleep apnoea, often do not know it. When they are asked about their sleep, they reply, "I sleep very well." Sleep specialists believe that obstructive sleep apnoea is very common and often not diagnosed. With sleep apnoea, the soft tissue in the throat or nose relaxes during sleep and blocks the airway, requiring extreme effort to breathe. The person struggles against the blockage for up to a minute, then wakes just long enough to gasp air, and falls back to sleep to start the cycle again. Unaware of waking dozens of times during the night, the person suffers from a lack of deep sleep, needed to restore the body's energy and work on the healing process. This, in turn leads to more symptoms such

as fatigue and pain. Sleep apnoea is a serious medical problem and can be life-threatening. It has been linked to heart disease and stroke and is believed to be the cause of death for many who die in their sleep from a heart attack. Sleep specialists suggest that people who are tired all the time in spite of a full night's sleep, or who find they need more sleep now than when they were younger, should be investigated for sleep apnoea or other sleep disorders, especially if they or their spouses report snoring.

Body and Mind

This chapter has outlined some causes for some common symptoms experienced by people with different chronic conditions. In addition it has suggested some things you can do to manage your symptoms. Taking physical action to deal with your physical symptoms is necessary for coping with your illness on a day-to-day basis, and can make a real difference to your comfort and your ability to cope.

You may benefit even further from taking time for yourself, with the intention of clearing your mind to gain a fresh perspective on your whole situation. The following chapter presents some ways to support your physical-symptom management with some conscious management of your mind. These are what are called cognitive techniques, which you can use to harness the power of your mind in the management of your condition. Your mind can help you reduce and even prevent some of the symptoms you may experience.

• • •

Suggested Further Reading

The Breathworks Project—mindfulness-based pain management and strategies for living well —may be worth investigating via the Internet.

Chalder, Trudie. *Coping with Chronic Fatigue*. London: Sheldon Press.

Dossey, Larry. *Prayer Is Good Medicine*. San Francisco: HarperCollins, 1996.

Farhi, Donna. *The Breathing Book: Vitality and Good Health Through Essential Breath Work.* Owl Books 1996

Gilbert, Paul. *Overcoming Depression.* Revised Ed. Constable Robinson, 2000.

Hanley, J.L. and Nancy Deville. *Tired of Being Tired.* London: Michael Joseph, 2002.

Hauck, Paul. *Calm Down.* London: Sheldon Press, 1980.

Johnston, Fiona. *Getting a Good Night's Sleep.* London: Sheldon Press, 2000.

Klein, Arthur C. *Chronic Pain— the Complete Guide to Relief.* Daily Telegraph Books Robinson Publishing, 2001

Santorelli, Saki. *Heal Thy Self -Lessons on Mindfulness in Medicine.* Random House/Bell Tower 1999

Shone, Neville. *Coping Successfully with Pain.* London: Sheldon Press, 2000.

Tannen, Deborah. *You Just Don't Understand: Men and Women in Conversation.* London: Virago, 1992.

Williams, Christopher J. *Overcoming Depression.* Sevenoaks, England: Arnold, 2001.

The material on pursed-lip, diaphragmatic and pursed-lip breathing was taken from the following two publications: *Essentials of Pulmonary Rehabilitation* by Thomas L. Petty, M.D., Brian Tiep, M.D., and Mary Burns, R.N., B.S. Pulmonary Education and Research Foundation, P.O. Box 1133, Lomita, CA 90717-5133; and *Help Yourself to Better Breathing*, American Lung Association, 1989.

CHAPTER
5

Using Your Mind To Manage Symptoms

Mind over matter?

There is a strong link between our thoughts, attitudes and emotions, and our mental and physical health. The expression "mind over matter" is often used to suggest that we can "rise above" physical sensations and situations if only we are strong enough. This makes the relationship between mind and body sound like a battle, which it is not, but the connection between the two is so close that we waste a powerful resource if we don't use our minds as part of our strategy to manage the physical experience of our lives.

Thoughts and emotions may not directly cause our chronic conditions, but they can influence the symptoms we experience. Hormones or other chemicals that carry messages throughout the body are triggered by what goes on in the mind. These messages affect how our body functions; for example, thoughts and emotions can change our heart rate, blood pressure, breathing, blood sugar levels, muscle responses, concentration, the ability to get pregnant, and our immune response to infection. What has been measured in laboratories is known to all of us from experience in our daily lives.

We have all experienced the power of the mind and its effects on the body. Pleasant and unpleasant thoughts create a bodily reaction. Our heart rate and breathing can increase or slow down; we may get cold sweats, hot sweats, blushing, tears, and so on. Crucially, just a memory or an image can create these physiological responses. When you really suck a real lemon, your body reacts in certain ways, but the important point, for understanding and using the techniques outlined in this chapter, is that the same physical reaction can subsequently be prompted by the *thought* of sucking a lemon.

Take a moment now and try this simple exercise. Imagine you are holding a big, bright yellow lemon. You hold it close to your nose and smell its strong citrus aroma. Now, you bite into the lemon. It's juicy! The juice fills your mouth and dribbles down your chin. Now you suck on the lemon and its tart juice.

What happens while this imaginary scene takes place? The body responds. Your mouth puckers and starts to water. You may even smell the scent of the lemon. All these clearly physical reactions are triggered by the mind and its memory of your experience with a real lemon.

We often take our imagination for granted. You may only now become aware of the mental control you have just exercised to imagine sucking the lemon. This chapter builds on our mental capacity to create images, to visualise pictures or scenes, and through those "imaginary" scenes, deliberately to change our physiological state.

Your mind has the power to affect your body so you can work on a mental level to manage physical symptoms associated with chronic conditions. With training and practice, you can use the mind to relax the body, to reduce stress and anxiety, and to ease physical and emotional discomfort. You may even be able to rely less on medication for symptom relief.

This chapter describes several ways of using your mind to manage symptoms. These are known as cognitive techniques. *Cognition* is the mental process of knowing, which includes such mental aspects as awareness, perception, reasoning, and judgment. So these techniques are usually referred to as cognitive techniques because they involve the use of thinking to make changes in the body.

Relaxation Techniques

We all have our own ways of relaxing. We may walk, watch TV, listen to music, knit, or garden. These familiar activities differ from the techniques that follow because they include some form of physical activity or require an external stimulus, like music. Taking a nap is also different because the mind isn't conscious; in the techniques discussed below, we use the mind actively to help the body achieve a relaxed state while awake.

The goal of relaxation is to "turn off" the outside world to allow the mind and body to rest. You can reduce tension and therefore reduce the intensity or severity of symptoms.

Basics for Starting Work on Using Your Mind

- Pick a place and time during the day when you won't be disturbed for fifteen minutes—start with five, if necessary, and if the only quiet room in the house is the bathroom, that'll do! Turn off the phone and make this time your own. Try to practise twice a day and four times a week.
- Don't expect miracles. It takes time to acquire skills. You may need three or four weeks of consistent practice before you really start to notice benefits.
- Relaxation should be helpful. At worst, you may find these few minutes boring, but if it is an unpleasant experience or makes you more nervous or anxious, then try one of the other symptom management techniques described in this chapter.

Muscle Relaxation

Muscle relaxation is one of the most commonly used cognitive techniques for symptom management. People like it because it makes sense. Muscular tension and physical stress intensifies pain, shortness of breath, or emotional distress, so releasing tension and stress can lessen those same symptoms. It is easy to learn. We can remember to use it in difficult situations. We can recognise some immediate positive results, in reduced pain, easier breathing and deeper calm. The results are lasting. It promotes restful sleep. So learning to use your mind to relax your muscles is worth some effort.

Below are three examples of muscle relaxation techniques with "scripts" to help you with the necessary thought processes. Look at the techniques and the scripts, try them, and choose one you like. You might want to tape-record a script, which can help you concentrate, without interruption from referring to the book.

You could buy your own relaxation tape or CD to use regularly. There are many available in shops and on the Internet. Ask about the return policy in case you find the tape or CD doesn't suit you.

The first script below helps you become familiar with the difference between how tension feels and how relaxation feels. The second script helps you scan your body, so that you can recognise where you are holding tension, and then release it. The script for the third muscle relaxation technique allows you direct access to your body's relaxation response.

Progressive Muscle Relaxation

Edmund Jacobson, an American physiologist from the last century, believed that once you learn to recognise the feeling of tension, you are better able to learn to let the tension go.

This first exercise introduces you to the technique for comparing the feelings of tension and relaxation. Pause for about ten seconds whenever there is a series of dots (. . .). Probably, just reading this script a couple of times and then working from memory will be enough. The exercise guides you through the major muscle groups, asking you first to tense and then to relax them. If you have a pain in a particular area today, tense those muscles only gently or not at all, and focus on relaxing them.

Progressive Muscle Relaxation Script

Take a few minutes for yourself, and let go of all outside concerns. Make yourself comfortable. Loosen tight clothing. Uncross your legs and ankles and let your arms and hands rest loosely on your knees. If you are lying, lie flat, perhaps with a book to raise your head slightly or a pillow under your knees to support you. Close your eyes.

Take a deep breath, filling your chest and breathing all the way down to the abdomen. Hold..... Breathe out through pursed lips, and, as you breathe out, let as much tension as possible flow out with your breath. Let all your muscles feel heavy and let your whole body just sink into the surface beneath you....

Become aware of the muscles in your feet and calves. Pull your toes back up toward your knees. Notice the tension .... Release and relax. ...Notice the discomfort leaving as relief and warmth replace it....

Now tighten the muscles of your thighs and buttocks. Hold and feel the tension... Let go and allow the muscles to relax. ...The relaxed muscles feel heavy and soft as if they're melting into the surface beneath you. ...

Tense the muscles in your abdomen and chest... Notice how you hold your breath as you tense. Relax, and notice that it is natural to want to take a deep breath to relieve the tension in this area... Take a deep breath now, breathing all the way down to the abdomen and letting the lower ribs, both front and back, expand ...As you breathe out, allow all the tension to flow out with your breath...

Now, stretching your fingers out straight, tense your fingers and tighten your arm muscles... Relax... Feel the tension flowing out as the circulation returns...

Press your shoulder blades together, tightening the muscles in your shoulders and neck...Many people carry tension here. Hold... Now, let go. Notice how the muscles feel warmer and more alive.

Tighten all the muscles of your face and head.. . Notice the tension, especially around your eyes and in your jaw... Now relax, allowing your jaw to become slack and slightly open... Notice the difference.

Now take another deep breath, breathing all the way down to the abdomen... And, as you breathe out, allow your body to sink heavily into the surface beneath you, and let any remaining tension flow out with the breath. ..You are becoming even more deeply relaxed...

Enjoy this comfortable feeling of relaxation.....

Prepare to come back to the here and now. Take three deep breaths. And, when you're ready, open your eyes.

Once you've practised this technique, you won't need to tense up parts of your body before you relax. You'll be aware of the area of tension and you'll able to let it go with a single deep breath. Remember the pleasant feeling as you let tension go. You can quieten your body and your mind like this.

For some people with a lot of pain, especially in the joints, the Jacobson technique may not be appropriate. If it hurts it may stop you relaxing, so don't tense those areas, just locate and release the tension. Or try another technique, like the body scan in the next script.

Body Scan

This is similar relaxation technique, which doesn't require the tensing or movement of muscles. Again, you can sit in a straight chair with your back supported, or you can lie down.

Body Scan Script

First, focus on your breathing. Spend a few minutes concentrating on each breath as it enters and leaves your body. Try directing your breath past your chest all the way down to your abdomen. This is diaphragmatic or belly breathing, which is described in chapter 4 and is an important part of all relaxation exercises.

After three or four minutes of concentrating on your breathing, move your attention to your toes. Don't move them, just think about how they feel. Don't worry if you don't feel anything at all. If you find any tension there, let it go as you breathe out.

After a few moments with your toes, move your attention to the bottoms of your feet. Again, don't move, just concentrate on any sensations you have. Let go of any tension you may find as you breathe out. Next, concentrate on the top of your feet and your ankles. After a few more moments, bring your attention to your lower legs.

Continue this process, shifting your attention every few moments to another part of your body, working slowly upwards to your head. If you find tension, let it go as you breathe out. If your mind wanders, just bring your attention back to your breathing and the feelings in your body.

There is likely to be tension in your shoulders, neck, jaw, face and scalp – don't neglect these. When you have finished, take three deep breaths and return your attention to the room.

You can use the body scan to help you get to sleep because it clears your mind of distracting thoughts. The key is to give your full attention to scanning your body for tension and releasing it.

The Relaxation Response

In the early 1970s, Dr Herbert Benson studied what he called "the relaxation response". He identified several natural states for our bodies. One "state" is the "fight or flight" response experienced by people faced with great danger. The body becomes tense, ready to fight or run away. This initial state of tension is followed naturally by the tendency to relax. This is the relaxation response. With the stresses and speed of many of our lives, our bodies are inclined to stay in a protracted or constant state of tension, and gradually we lose our ability to relax. To elicit the relaxation response, we can practise the following exercise.

Again find your quiet place. Allow about twenty minutes. You will need to choose a word, such as "one", an object, like a flower, or a pleasant feeling, such as "peace", to focus on. Expect the experience to be a positive one. Let yourself be. Thoughts, images and feelings will float into your consciousness. Just allow them, passively, to float out again as you bring your mind back to your chosen focus.

Relaxation Response Script

Sit quietly in a comfortable position.

Close your eyes.

Relax all your muscles, starting at your feet and working up to your face. Keep them relaxed.

Breathe in through your nose. Become aware of your breathing. As you breathe out through your mouth, say the word you chose silently to yourself. Try to empty all thoughts from your mind; concentrate on your word.

Continue this for ten to twenty minutes. You may open your eyes to check the time but don't use an alarm. When you finish, sit quietly for several minutes, keeping your eyes closed. Don't stand up for a few minutes.

Don't worry about whether you have achieved a deep level of relaxation. Keep a passive attitude and let relaxation occur at its own pace. When you get distracting thoughts, just bring your attention gently back to repeating the word you chose.

Practise this once or twice a day, but leave two hours after a meal. Digestion can get in the way of relaxation.

This exercise is very much like meditation, which is discussed later in this chapter.

Using Your Imagination

You can reduce fear and anxiety and refocus your attention away from the discomfort of your symptoms using your imagination. Techniques include guided imagery and visualisation.

Guided Imagery

The guided-imagery relaxation technique uses your powerful imaginative capacity—as in the example with the lemon above. Allowing yourself to wander in the world your imagination creates from the script is like being guided through a daydream. You can divert your attention from your symptoms and transport yourself to another time and place. You can achieve deep relaxation in your body by picturing yourself in a peaceful environment.

The guided-imagery script presented here can help take you on a mental stroll. Again, you can read the script several times so that you know what it says. You could ask a family member or a friend to read you the script slowly, pausing for about ten seconds when there is a series of dots (….).Or you could make a tape recording of the script and play it to yourself. This has the advantage that your own voice takes you on your "guided tour".

Again, make yourself as comfortable as possible, sitting or lying down. Loosen any tight clothing. Uncross your arms, legs and ankles. Allow your body to feel completely supported by the surface on which you are sitting or lying. Close your eyes.

Guided Imagery Script: A Walk in the Country

Take a deep breath in through your nose, breathing all the way down to the abdomen. Hold....Breathe out slowly through slightly pursed lips, and, as you do, relax your whole body, allowing all your muscles to feel limp and heavy....

Scan your body for any muscle tension, starting with your head and passing all the way down to your toes...

Release any tension in your face, head and neck by letting your jaw become slack and your head feel heavy on your shoulders. ..Allow your shoulders to drop heavily... Take a deep breath and relax your chest and abdomen. ...Allow your arms and legs to feel heavy and to sink into the surface beneath you...

Now take a deep breath and become aware of any remaining tension in your body... As you breathe out, allow all the muscles of your body to sink heavily into the surface beneath you, becoming even more deeply relaxed....

Imagine yourself walking along an old country lane...there are trees beside the lane...you move from sunlight to dappled shade, and back to sunlight....the sun is warm on your back...the birds are singing.

Soon, you have come to a wooden gate in the hedge. Open it. The wood is rough on your hands ... you go through, turning to lift the gate shut behind you... You find yourself in a meadow in full sunlight. Soft green grasses... Flowers growing where they've seeded themselves . . . honeysuckle growing in the hedgerow. . . . Breathe deeply, smelling the flowers, the sweet clean air... Listen to the birds and insects. Feel the gentle breeze warm against your skin. . . . Close your eyes and turn your face to the sun, it glows red through your eyelids. ..All your senses are alive and responding with pleasure to this peaceful time and place.

When you're ready to move on, you slowly follow a path, step after step after step... Now there are trees and you walk between them... The sun is filtered through the leaves... The air feels soft and a little cooler...

Listen... You become aware of the sound of a nearby stream... You can smell it... You pause, breathing in deeply the cool and fragrant air several times, and with each breath you feel more refreshed... Soon, you come to the stream. It is clear and clean as it flows and tumbles over rocks... There are fallen logs, with moss...the brightest green... the water swirls around them and gushes sparkling past you...

You follow a path beside the stream for a little way...There are trunks of trees around you... You look up and you can see the blue of the sky through the leaves of the high branches. You come out into a sunlit clearing... there is a small waterfall emptying over a rough grey rock into a quiet pool of water. ..You see red, orange, yellow... a rainbow, in the mist.

You find a comfortable place on a soft green bank to sit for a while. ..You can reach the water with your fingertips... A perfect place where you can feel utterly relaxed... You are part of the warmth and light of this peaceful place ...and you are completely content...

After a while, you become aware that it's time to return... You walk back down the path through the cool and fragrant trees, out into the sun-drenched meadow, one last smell of the flowers and out through the gate onto the lane.

You leave this secret retreat for now and walk slowly back down the lane... You feel calm and rested. You know that you can visit your special place whenever you wish to take some time to refresh yourself and renew your energy.

Be aware of your body, again, relaxed and easy... When you are ready to, take three deep breaths and open your eyes.

Visualisation

This technique is similar to guided imagery. It is another way to use your imagination to create a picture of yourself doing things you want to do. We all use a form of visualisation every day, without realising it – when we dream, worry, read a book, or listen to a story. In all these activities the mind creates images for us to "see". We also use visualisation intentionally when we make plans for the day, consider the possible outcomes of a decision we have to make, or rehearse for an event or an activity. Our minds can manage visualisations even while we are doing something else.

You can, as with the lemon memory above, use pleasant scenes from your past for visualisations. To practise this, you might try to remember every detail of a special holiday or party that made you happy. Who was there? What happened? What did you do or talk about? You can also use visualisation to create your own images, new scenes, which is where this technique differs from guided imagery where the images are suggested to you. New scenes could include planning for some future event, or filling in the details of a fantasy. How would you spend a million pounds? What would your ideal home or garden look like? What would you do for your holiday of a lifetime?

You can use your mind to visualise symbols to represent the pain or discomfort felt in a part of your body. For example, a painful joint might be red or a tight chest might be visualised as having a tight band round it. Once you have an image, you can use the power of your mind to change it. The red colour fades away, leaving a healthy pink or the tight band might stretch and stretch until it falls off leaving the chest free. By deliberately formulating images which accurately represent your symptom, you make it possible to work mentally to change those images. Then the new images allow your perception of the pain or the discomfort to change. This can require some perseverance but, again, it is worth the discipline of practising for a few minutes as often as you can manage. Individuals have found in their own lives that the technique has helped them actually reduce the discomfort of symptoms through changing the imagery associated with them.

Visualisation helps build confidence and skill so it is useful for setting and accomplishing your personal goals and action planning - see chapter 2. Use visualisation when you are writing your action plan, and afterwards, take a few minutes to visualise the detail of yourself taking the walk, doing the exercises, or eating a plate of carefully chosen food. Here you are mentally rehearsing the steps on the way to your goals. The more precise the visualisation, the more real the scene will seem. Numerous scientific studies have shown that this technique can help people to master skills and to reach personal targets.

All the relaxation techniques mentioned above can be used in conjunction with diaphragmatic breathing. This breathing technique is described in detail in chapter 4. It can help you achieve a more relaxed state which facilitates all the mental exercises in this chapter.

Other Cognitive Strategies

Learning to relax is an important part of symptom management, but other cognitive strategies can also be useful. These techniques, developing other aspects of your mental skills, may require more practice than learning muscle relaxation, before you notice the benefits, but they are worth the effort. They include distraction, positive thinking or self-talk, meditation, and prayer.

Distraction

We are usually aware of a great many things in our surroundings, but our minds have trouble focusing on more than one thing at a time. This has the advantage for us, that, if we train our minds to focus attention on something other than our bodies and their sensations, we can lessen the intensity of our physical symptoms. The technique of distraction—attention refocusing—is particularly helpful for people who feel their symptoms are overwhelming, or who worry that every bodily sensation might be a sign that their condition is getting worse.

Distraction trains your mind to move its attention away from your symptoms. It does not mean that you ignore the symptoms, but that you choose not to dwell on them. It works well for short activities or for times when you know your symptoms will be a problem. You might try one of the following distraction techniques.

Really involve yourself in what you are doing. For instance, if you are washing up, play the radio at the same time or a favourite CD. Use a washing up liquid with a smell you really like, or use an essential oil. Really concentrate on the warmth and feel of the water as you pull your hands through it. Concentrating on what you are doing leaves less space in your brain to feel symptoms.

Focus on what you will do after whatever it is you don't like doing. For example, if climbing stairs is painful, think about what you will do when you get to the top. If sleep is slow to come, decide not to think about that but sort out the details for some future event.

Play games in your head—think of a person's name, say, for every letter of the alphabet. If you get stuck on one letter go on to the next. Count backwards in threes from 100 (100, 97, 94…). Imagine your floor is a map of the world, if vacuuming or sweeping causes you problems. As you move across the area, try naming all the countries moving east to west or north to south. If you are not very good at geography, imagine your favourite shopping centre and where each shop is to be found. Remember the words to your favourite songs or all the characters in your favourite TV soap opera or film. You can simply take your mind off whatever is causing you difficulty or discomfort, by deciding to focus it on something else. There are, of course, a million variations to these examples.

So far, this chapter has suggested short-term strategies, refocusing your mind internally on something other than your physical symptoms. But you can also deliberately make distraction work the other way round, by choosing what you do physically to take your mind off problems - for example, depression and some forms of chronic pain. Commit your time to an activity or hobby or job that interests you - cooking, reading, home study, going to the cinema, maybe even volunteering to help other people. Enjoying what you are doing engages your mind. Keeping yourself interested is a great self-management skill. It takes courage, decisiveness, action planning and organisation. And it rewards you with huge dividends. One of the marks of a successful self-manager is that they have a variety of interests and always seem to be doing something rewarding.

Positive Thinking and Self-Talk

We all talk to ourselves a lot of the time. We think in words things like, "I'm so tired, I don't want to cook tonight." Or "I'm so glad I saw that film last night, it was such fun". What we think and then say to ourselves is called 'self-talk'. The tone and content of our self-talk tends to come from how and what we think about ourselves. Our thoughts can be positive or negative, strengthening or destructive, and so is our self-talk. . Therefore, self-talk can be an important self-management tool. You can learn to make self-talk work for you by keeping it positive.

Our self-talk is learned from the way others have spoken to us—sometimes, unfortunately, negatively—and it becomes part of us as we grow up. Negative self-talk might include remarks that begin with something like: "I just can't do…" "If only I could…" If only I didn't…" "It's not fair…" "I don't have the energy…" "How could I be so stupid?" This type of self-talk represents our doubts and fears about ourselves and our ability to deal with our condition and its symptoms. Just as if it were someone else saying it to us, it damages our self-esteem, attitude, and mood. Negative self-talk makes us feel bad and our symptoms worse.

What we say to ourselves affects our success in becoming good self-managers. If we keep being told—even if it's our own self talking—that we can't cope, can't learn, can't change, then we'll tend to believe it and make it come true. If we repeatedly hear you can, you're clever, you did well, we'll feel different and behave differently. Luckily we can assess what we think, and choose what to say. Either we can tell ourselves negative things, limit our abilities and actions, and become prisoners of our negative statements. Or, we can choose to tell ourselves positive things. We can learn new, healthier, kinder and encouraging ways to think about ourselves, so that our self-talk can work for us instead of against us. By changing negative, defeatist statements to positive ones, we can manage our symptoms much more effectively.

Changing the way you think needs practice and takes time, because you may very well be changing the habits literally of a lifetime. But if you would rather have a kind, encouraging voice talking you through your days, you can.

Think about the following steps:

- Listen carefully to what you say to yourself or about yourself. Write down all the negative self-talk statements, especially during times that are particularly difficult for you. For example, what do you say to yourself when you get up in the morning with pain, while doing the exercises you don't really like, or at the times you are feeling low? Challenge the negative thoughts by asking yourself questions to sort out why you believe this, and what, if anything, about the statement is really true. For example, are you exaggerating the situation, generalising, worrying too much, assuming the worst? Maybe you are making an unrealistic or unfair comparison, assuming too much responsibility, taking something too personally, or expecting perfection. Look at the evidence and go to the next step of establishing the positive.
- Work on finding a positive statement to replace each negative statement you identified. The positive statements can be called affirmations. Write these down. Positive statements will reflect your decision to be in control. So, lying in bed in the morning, your new self-talk might be "I want to get up now because I like getting ready without rushing" or "I'm feeling better this morning and that means I can get a bit further with the job I began yesterday" or "People like me and I like me too".

- Read and rehearse the affirmations you have arrived at, either privately or with another person. Try saying them to your image in the mirror! Consciously repeating positive self-talk will help you notice and throw out the worn-out negative thoughts.
- Practise the new affirmative statements in real situations. Taking time to practise will let you develop new positive thinking patterns which are quite automatic.

Changing even a single negative thought to positive self-talk makes a difference. As new positive self-talk influences all your thinking, it will be a powerful tool in your self-management programme. You can use it to manage your symptoms and your situation. It will help you also to master the other skills discussed in this book. It's a technique worth putting your mind to.

Prayer and Meditation

Religious and spiritual beliefs are vital to many people. Beliefs bring a sense of meaning and purpose to life, and help us put things into perspective and set priorities. They may help us find comfort in difficult times. They can motivate us to make necessary changes. Even if we aren't supported by membership of a particular church or religious group, we very likely operate on a set of beliefs.

Recent medical and scientific research suggests that maintaining religious or spiritual beliefs may improve health. People who belong to a religious or spiritual community, or who regularly pray or meditate, have better health and live longer than those who do not. One explanation could be that prayer and meditation help increase people's emotional well-being by giving strength and a sense of control – positively affecting the body. Perhaps seeing their situation in the broader context provided by religion allows people to be happier. Maybe religious or spiritual beliefs encourage a healthy lifestyle. Possibly the support people tend to receive from membership of a group improves their health.

We know from scientifically conducted trials in a laboratory situation that people experience the relaxation response when they pray or meditate. Their blood pressure, heart rate, and levels of stress hormones drop. At the same time, the brain waves associated with relaxation increase. These physiological changes reduce anxiety and increase blood protein levels in the body, indicating a healthier immune system. Prayer and meditation also provide a form of distraction for people with long-term health conditions. They are able to refocus their attention away from their symptoms, thereby reducing the intensity of the discomfort caused by those symptoms.

Regardless of the rationale, prayer and meditation remain the oldest of self-management tools and are practised in all parts of the world. While these cannot be "prescribed" for you, it might be very productive for you to explore your own beliefs. If you are religious, try practising prayer and meditation more consistently. If you are not religious, you might consider adopting some form of meditation or reflection—as suggested below—for regular practice.

Centring Prayer

All the major religions of the world use some form of prayer. Basically, prayer is talking with and listening to your God, a way to spend time with your God, putting yourself in the hands of your God and expressing or sharing your feelings, wants and needs. Prayer can be done publicly with others or privately at home. You might pray to give thanks and praise, to ask for help or forgiveness. There are many kinds of prayer, but there is one form, in particular, that can produce positive effects in your daily life. This is called the centring prayer and is very similar to some types of meditation.

Choose a sacred or special word—something like *Lord, Father, Mother, Abba, Omm, love, peace, shalom* to express your intention for the centring prayer. Set aside at least twenty minutes of quiet time. A full stomach can make you drowsy, so avoid meal-times. Find a quiet, comfortable place to sit, keeping your back straight and closing your eyes. Let go of whatever is going on. Gently introduce and focus on your sacred word. Do not focus on other thoughts that drift into your mind, just return to your sacred word. At the end of your prayer period, remain in silence with your eyes closed for a couple of minutes.

During your prayer, you may notice physical sensations, like slight pains, itches, or twitches in parts of your body as your body releases both its physical and emotional tension. There may be either a heaviness or lightness in your arms and legs. When this happens, just allow yourself to notice the sensations briefly, and return to your sacred word.

Start with once a day but aim to practise the centring prayer twice each day. Over time, you will experience positive results in your life.

Mindfulness Meditation

There are many approaches to meditation but its central purpose is to quieten the mind. Through this, it can help quieten the body. So it is a useful technique for people with long-term conditions, to help manage pain, stress, tiredness or shortness of breath. Mindfulness meditation can be practised by anyone. It is quite simple. All you need is a quiet place and about five minutes. You can sit in a chair with your feet flat on the ground and your hands in your lap or on your knees, or sit on the floor with legs crossed in a more traditional yoga position. It does not matter so long as you are comfortable.

The essence of mindfulness meditation is to concentrate on your breathing. It is best if you can do diaphragmatic or belly breathing, but you do not have to take deep breaths. The main thing is to keep your full attention on your breathing. Breathe in slowly, hold your breath for a moment; then breathe out slowly. At all times, concentrate on your breathing.

While the procedure is very simple, you will find that your mind easily wanders. It is full of chatter—some people call this "having a monkey mind". As soon as you notice your mind wandering, simply bring your attention back to your breathing. At first you may only manage a minute or two but your attention will improve with practice.

You may become uncomfortably aware of a part of your body during meditation. When this happens, do nothing but pay attention to your breathing. In many cases, you will find that the discomfort goes away. If it continues, however, scratch the itch or change the position, but as you do this, pay full attention to what you are doing – be mindful of it. With mindfulness meditation it is important to be fully aware of what you are doing at that moment.

Like the other techniques for managing your symptoms through your mind, mindfulness meditation requires practice. It is unlikely (but not impossible!) that you will see results immediately. But—with practice—five minutes a day at first, building to fifteen to thirty minutes a day, four or five times a week, this can be a very effective symptom management tool.

"Don't just do something—sit there!"

In Conclusion: Some Key Principles of Symptom Self-Management So Far

Symptoms of long-term conditions, their causes and the ways they interact are complex. A vicious circle can be set up in people's daily lives, which requires decision and effort to break. Understanding the nature, causes and interactions of symptoms will make management easier.

Self-managers work to identify symptoms, isolate possible causes and effects, and take action to break the cycle. There is more than one way to manage most symptoms. Not all management techniques work for everyone. Each self-manager undertakes to experiment and find out what works best for them.

Trying different techniques can be done systematically via action-planning, monitoring the results to see what works.

Learning new skills and taking control can take time. Practice is important for mastering any skill. Using the mind to manage a health condition requires time and practice.

"Stickability" matters! Perseverance pays!

• • •

Suggested Further Reading

Chalder, Trudie. *Coping with Chronic Fatigue*. London: Sheldon Press.

Hanley, J.L. and Nancy Deville. *Tired of Being Tired*. London: Michael Joseph, 2002.

Hauck, Paul. *Calm Down*. London: Sheldon Press, 1980.

Johnston, Fiona. *Getting a Good Night's Sleep*. London: Sheldon Press, 2000.

Ornstein, Robert, and David Sobel. *Healthy Pleasures*. Reading, Mass.: Addison-Wesley, 1990.

Shone, Neville. *Coping Successfully with Pain*. London: Sheldon Press, 2000.

Tannen, Deborah. *You Just Don't Understand: Men and Women in Conversation*. London: Virago, 1992.

Williams, Christopher J. *Overcoming Depression*. Sevenoaks, England: Arnold, 2001.

CHAPTER 6

Exercising for Fun and Fitness

"The weakest and oldest among us can become some sort of athlete, but only the strongest can survive as spectators. Only the hardiest can withstand the perils of inertia, inactivity, and immobility."

Regular exercise and physical activity are vital to our physical and emotional health and can bring fun and fitness at the same time. This can be hard to remember with a chronic illness, and growing older can also make an active lifestyle seem far away. Some people have never been very active and others have given up leisure activities because of illness.

The truth is that long periods of inactivity in anyone, young or old, ill or well, can lead to weakness, stiffness, fatigue, poor appetite, high blood pressure, obesity, osteoporosis, constipation, and increased sensitivity to pain, anxiety, and depression. Because symptoms like these also arise from chronic illnesses, it can be difficult to tell whether it is the illness, the inactivity, or a combination of the two that is responsible for these problems. Chapter 1 showed the need to sort out carefully the causes and the effects of symptoms, in order to work out an action plan to deal with them. We don't yet have cures for all the illnesses which can cause these symptoms, but luckily we know exactly what to do about inactivity – be active! Exercise!

Most of us would agree in theory that exercising and being active is healthier and more satisfying than being inactive. However, when it comes to putting that theory into practice, we are brought up short because we don't know exactly what to do, and we don't even know who to ask for help. Programmes in books and on videos don't seem to apply to us, and it can be frightening to launch on a new activity without knowing exactly what is possible and what is safe for us.

Thanks to the knowledge gained from many people with chronic illnesses who have worked with health professionals in exercise research, there is now reliable information available to guide us. This book draws on the experience of people whose situations have much in common, even if their conditions have different names. Using the information in the three chapters on exercise, it is possible to make informed action plans to exercise for fun and fitness, for flexibility and strength, and for endurance.

Sometimes exercise programmes collapse because we lose sight of their overall purpose. What we do each day doesn't seem to provide immediate results, although most people would say that they do feel better just for having done something that day. It can be hard to keep on finding the motivation. But with our clearly formulated goal of self-management, we can keep reminding ourselves that this bit of exercise, today, is a step on the road to taking control. We can help ourselves manage symptoms and make everyday activities less stressful and more enjoyable

This chapter will help you to improve your health and fitness and make wise exercise choices. What your health professional has advised you already still applies - the information in these chapters is not intended to take the place of professional therapeutic recommendations. If you've had an exercise plan prescribed for you that differs from the suggestions here, take this book to your doctor or physiotherapist and ask what they think about this programme. Sometimes, health professionals prescribe exercise programmes that don't take into account people's personal circumstances or preferences. If this is the case for you, you may wish to talk this through with your health professional, perhaps referring to the chapter 9 Communicating for extra ideas.

Regular exercise benefits everyone, but especially people with chronic health problems. Regular exercise makes you stronger, less anxious and more cheerful. Exercise can help maintain a good weight, which takes stress off weight-bearing joints and improves blood pressure, blood sugar and blood fat levels. There is evidence that regular exercise can help to "thin" the blood, or prevent blood clots, which is one of the reasons exercise can be of particular benefit to people with heart disease, cerebrovascular disease, and peripheral vascular disease.

In addition, strong muscles can help people with arthritis to protect their joints by improving stability and absorbing shock. Regular exercise also helps nourish joints and keep cartilage and bone healthy. Regular exercise has been shown to help people with chronic lung disease improve endurance and reduce shortness of breath—and the number of trips to Accident and Emergency departments. Many people with claudication - leg pain from severe atherosclerotic constriction in the arteries of the lower extremities - can walk farther without leg pain after undertaking a regular exercise programme. Studies of people with heart disease who exercise in cardiac rehabilitation programmes suggest that exercise may even increase life expectancy. Regular exercise is an important part of controlling blood sugar levels, losing weight, and reducing the risks of cardiovascular complications for people with diabetes.

Many people with long term medical conditions find that starting exercise can be quite tough. Some people find that their symptoms are initially made a little worse. Getting the body going again can cause the body to complain a little; it hasn't been used to exercise! The key seems to be not to give up, but to start with small steps (in the most literal way) and to build up over time. Develop goals and an action plan.

The good news is that it doesn't take hours of painful, sweat-soaked exercise to achieve most of these health benefits. Even short periods of gentle physical activity can significantly improve your health and fitness, reduce disease risks, and give your mood a boost.

Exercise reconditions your body, helping you to do much of what you did before you were ill and became less mobile. This will help you improve your health, feel better, and manage your chronic illness. Feeling more in control and less at the mercy of your chronic illness is one of the biggest and best benefits of becoming an exercise self-manager.

Developing an Active Lifestyle

Right, so you want to be more physically active. Well done, already! You can set aside a special time for a formal exercise programme, involving such planned activities as walking, jogging, swimming, tennis, aerobic dance, exercise to an exercise videotape, and so on. But don't underestimate the value and importance of just being more physically active throughout the day as you carry out your usual activities. Both can be helpful.

The formal programmes are usually more visible and get more attention. But being more physical in everyday life can also pay off. Consider taking the stairs a floor or two instead of waiting impatiently for a lift. When travelling to work or going shopping by car, park several hundred yards away and walk the remaining distance, rather than trying to find a nearby parking space. Mow the lawn, work in the garden, or just get up once in a while and walk around the house.

These types of daily activities, often not viewed as "exercise," can add up to significant health benefits. Recent studies show that even small amounts of daily activity can raise fitness levels, decrease heart disease risk, and positively alter mood, and the activities can be pleasurable, enjoyable ones! Playing with the children, dancing, gardening, bowls, golf - all these enjoyable activities can make a big difference. One person commented that she never exercised. When asked why she went line dancing several times a week she replied, "Oh, that's not exercise, that's fun." The average day is filled with excellent opportunities to be more physical.

Developing an Exercise Programme

For many people, however, a more formal exercise programme can be helpful. This usually involves setting aside a period of time, several times a week, to deliberately focus on increasing fitness. A complete, balanced exercise programme should help you improve these three aspects of fitness:

1. **Flexibility.** This refers to the ability of the joints and muscles to move comfortably through a full, normal range of motion. Limited flexibility can cause pain, increase risk of injury, and make muscles less efficient. Flexibility tends to diminish with inactivity, age, and certain conditions, but you can increase or maximise your flexibility by doing gentle stretching exercises like those described later in Chapter 7.

2. **Strength.** Muscles need to be exercised to maintain their strength. If we don't move enough, our muscles tend to weaken and shrink. The weaker the muscles get, the less we feel like using them, and the more inactive we tend to become, creating a vicious circle. Much of the disability and lack of mobility for people with chronic illness is due to muscle weakness. You can reverse this weakness with a programme of gradually increasing exercise.

3. **Endurance.** Our ability to keep an activity going depends on certain vital capacities. The heart and lungs must work efficiently to distribute oxygen-rich blood to the muscles. The muscles must be conditioned to use the oxygen.

Aerobic exercise, which means exercise "with oxygen", improves cardiovascular and muscular conditioning. This type of exercise uses the large muscles of your body in a rhythmical, continuous activity. The most effective activities involve your whole body - walking, swimming, dancing, mowing the lawn, and so on. Aerobic exercise improves cardiovascular fitness, lessens heart attack risk and helps control weight. It promotes a sense of well-being - easing depression and anxiety, promoting restful sleep, and improving mood and energy levels.

Your Fitness Programme

To be "fit" implies being "fit" for something. Someone contemplating climbing Everest requires to be fit for that. Most of us don't. Generally if we are fit for what we want to do plus a bit extra, we will feel better. Of course, as we do more, so our general level of fitness can and does go up, and we want to do more—the opposite of the "vicious circle" that has been described before. Exercises like those in these three chapters are designed to move us on from wherever we are now. So a complete fitness programme combines exercises to improve each of the three aspects of fitness: flexibility, strength, and endurance. Chapter 7 explains and illustrates a number of flexibility and strengthening exercises. Chapter 8 contains information about endurance or aerobic exercise. If you haven't exercised regularly in some time, or have pain, stiffness, shortness of breath, or weakness that interferes with your daily activities, it is a good idea to discuss your ideas about increasing your exercise with health professionals. Begin your fitness programme by choosing a number of flexibility and strengthening exercises that you are willing to do every day or every other day. Once you are able to comfortably exercise for at least ten minutes at a time, you are ready to start adding some endurance or aerobic activities.

Many people wonder how to choose the right exercises and how to know what's best for them. The truth is that the best exercises for you are the ones that will help you do what you want to do. Often, the most important decision to start a successful fitness programme is to choose a goal (something you want to do) that exercise can help you reach. You might like to re-read the section in chapter 2 on action-planning. Once you have a goal in mind, it is much easier to choose exercises that make sense to you. There is no doubt that we all are more successful exercisers if we know where we want exercise to take us. If you don't see how exercise can be helpful to you, it is hard to get excited about adding just another task to our days.

Choose your goal and make your action plan:

1. **Choose a goal that you want to reach but don't or can't do now because of some physical reason.** For example, you might

want to enjoy a shopping or fishing expedition with your friends, mow the lawn, or take a family holiday.

2. **Think about why you can't or don't do it or enjoy doing it now.** It might be that you get tired before everybody else, that it's too hard to get up from a low chair or bench, that climbing steps is painful or makes your legs tired, or that your shoulders are too weak or stiff to cast your fishing line or carry a heavy bag.

3. **Decide what about your abilities makes it difficult to do what you want.** For example, if getting up from a low seat is difficult, you may realise that your hips, knees, or joints are stiff and that your leg muscles are weak. In this case, look for flexibility and strengthening exercises for hips and knees. If you decide a major problem is that your shoulders are stiff and your arms too weak to handle a heavy bag, choose flexibility and strengthening exercises for your shoulders and arms.

4. **Design your exercise plan.** Choose no more than 10–12 exercises at first. Start by doing 3–5 repetitions of each and review the information in chapter 7. As you get comfortable, you can increase repetitions and kinds of exercise. If you want to improve your endurance, read over chapter 8 about aerobic exercise. Start off with short periods and build up gradually. Health and fitness take time to build, but every day you exercise you are healthier and on your way to fitness. That's why it's so important to make sure you keep it up. Keeping a journal—or just a list on a calendar of which exercises you did and how often—can help you apply the problem-solving steps from chapter 2, if you find you need to modify your programme after trying it out for a couple of weeks.

What Are Your Exercise Barriers?

Health and fitness make sense. Yet, when faced with actually doing something, most people can come up with scores of excuses, concerns and worries. These barriers can prevent us from even taking the first step. Here are some common barriers and possible solutions:

- **"I don't have enough time."** Everyone has the same amount of time. We just choose to use it differently. It's a matter of priorities.

Some find a lot of time for television, but nothing to spare for fitness. It doesn't really take a lot of time. Even five minutes a day is a good start, and it's much better than no physical activity. You may be able to combine activities, like watching television while pedalling a stationary bicycle, or arranging "walking meetings" to discuss business or family matters.

- **"I'm too tired."** When you're out of shape, you feel listless and tend to tire easily. Then you don't exercise because you're tired, and this becomes yet another vicious circle. You have to break out of the "too tired" cycle. Regular physical activity increases your stamina and gives you more energy to do the things you like. As you get back into shape, you will recognise the difference between feeling listless or "out of shape" and feeling physically tired.
- **"I'm too old."** You're never too old for some type of physical activity. No matter what your level of fitness is or your age, you can always find some ways to increase activity, energy, and sense of well-being. Fitness is especially important as we age.
- **"I'm too ill."** It may be true that you are too ill for a vigorous or strenuous exercise programme, but you can usually find some ways to be more active. Remember, you can exercise one minute at a time, several times a day. The enhanced physical fitness can help you better cope with your illness and prevent further problems.
- **"I get enough exercise."** This may be true, but for most people, their jobs and daily activities don't provide enough sustained exercise to keep them fully fit and energetic.
- **"Exercise is boring."** You can make it more interesting and fun. Exercise with other people. Entertain yourself with a headset and audio tapes or listen to the radio. Vary your activities and your walking routes.
- **"Exercise is painful."** The old saying "No pain, no gain" is simply wrong and out-of-date. Recent evidence shows that significant health benefits come from gentle, low-intensity, enjoyable physical activity. You may sweat, or feel a bit short of breath, but if you feel more pain when you finish than before you started, take a

close look at what you are doing. More likely than not, you are either exercising improperly or overdoing it for your particular condition. Talk to your instructor, physiotherapist or doctor. You may simply need to be less vigorous or change the type of exercise that you're doing.

- **"I'm too embarrassed."** For some, the thought of putting on a skintight, "designer" exercise outfit and prancing around in public is delightful, but for others it is downright distressing. Fortunately, as we'll describe, the options for physical activity range from exercise in the privacy of your own home to group social activities. You should be able to find something that suits you.
- **"I'm afraid I might fall."** Many people who are afraid of falling, or who have fallen, decide to limit activity in order to avoid falls. This might seem to make sense in the short term, but before long, inactivity and the weakness and stiffness that result from it can actually increase the risk of falling. Maintaining strong and flexible legs and ankles, and staying active so that you practise balancing in different positions are important to reduce the risk of falls. If your balance worries you, be sure to read the next section "Improving Balance"; also look in chapter 7 for the balance exercises marked "BB" and the exercises 26-31 at the end of the exercise section.
- **"I'm afraid I'll have a heart attack."** In most cases, the risk of a heart attack may be greater for those who are not physically active than for those who exercise regularly. If you are worried about this, consult your doctor, but for people whose illness is under control, it's probably safer to exercise than not to exercise.
- **"It's too cold, it's too hot, it's too dark," and so on.** If you are adaptable, and vary your type of exercise, you can generally work around the changes in weather that make certain types of exercise more difficult. Consider indoor activities like using an exercise bicycle or walking through a museum or shopping centre.
- **"I'm afraid I won't be able to do it right. I'm afraid I'll fail."** Many people don't start a new project because they are afraid they won't succeed. If you feel this way about starting an exercise programme, remember two things. Firstly, whatever activities you are able to do—no matter how short or "easy"—will be much better for you than doing nothing. Be proud of what you have done, not

guilty about what you haven't done. Use positive self-talk to congratulate yourself. Secondly, new projects often seem overwhelming—until we get started and learn to enjoy each day's adventures and successes.

Perhaps you have come up with some other barriers. The human mind is incredibly creative! But you can turn that creativity to your advantage by using it to refute the excuses and develop positive attitudes about exercise and fitness. If you get stuck, ask others for suggestions, or try some of the self-talk suggestions in chapter 5.

Improving Balance

It is common for people who become weak or who have been inactive for some time to have poorer balance and to worry about falling. Too often, people decide that the best way not to fall is to spend more time sitting and not doing anything active. You might think that if you are not up walking around, you won't be at risk of falling down, the effects of being inactive are weakness, stiffness, slower reflexes and slower muscles. All these actually harm your ability to balance and will eventually increase your risk of falling.

Falls can be caused by personal conditions such as weakness, dizziness, stiffness, poor eyesight, medication effects, loss of sensation, or inner ear problems. Falls can also be caused by external conditions such as poor lighting, uneven surfaces, rugs and carpets, and cluttered floors. Your ability to avoid falls depends on reducing the environmental risks and keeping yourself strong, flexible, and capable of staying upright even when something gets in your way or puts you off balance. Research shows that people who have strong legs and ankles, who are flexible and who practise activities that require them to maintain and recover their balance, have less fear of falling and actually fall less. If you have fallen or are afraid that you may fall, it is a good idea to talk with your doctor, get your balance checked to make sure there are no vision or inner ear problems to be addressed, and look critically at your home with health and safety in mind. Exercising to keep yourself strong, flexible, and active also helps protect you from falling.

Preparing to Exercise

Working out how to make the commitment of time and energy to regular exercise is a challenge for everyone, even more so if you have a chronic illness. You'll need to find a comfortable programme and take sensible precautions to make sure you're safe. But you can be confident that even with a chronic illness, most people can do some kind of aerobic exercise.

If your illness is not fairly stable, if you have been inactive for more than six months, if you have a heart condition, or if you have questions about starting an aerobic exercise programme, it is best to use one of your professional consultants, perhaps your doctor or physiotherapist who have more specialist knowledge than you have. Take this book with you when you discuss your exercise ideas, and prepare a list of your specific questions, because for self-management, you need to be able to decide what's best for you, on the basis of all the information you can gather.

Part of responsible self-management is learning how much to push your exercising, without doing "too much." Be alert to the symptoms of your own particular condition and find out which ones you should not "exercise through". If a problem comes up, speak to your doctor about it, and begin exercising again only after getting the doctor's clearance to do so. Also, don't exercise when you are experiencing flu symptoms, an upset stomach, diarrhoea, or other acute illnesses.

So, start by learning your individual needs and limits. If possible, talk to your doctor and other health professionals who understand your kind of chronic illness. Listen to their ideas about special exercise needs and precautions. Learn to be aware of your body, and then get on with your action plan.

Respect your body. Do your warm-up, and if you can't comfortably complete your warm-up period of flexibility and strengthening exercises, then don't try to do more vigorous conditioning exercises. Your personal exercise programme should be based on your current level of health and fitness, your goals and desires, your abilities and special needs, and your likes and dislikes. Deciding to improve your fitness, and feeling the satisfaction of success, has nothing to do with competition or comparing yourself to others, so take it steady.

Opportunities In Your Community

Most people who exercise regularly do so with at least one other person. Two or more people can keep each other motivated, and a whole class can build a feeling of camaraderie. On the other hand, exercising alone gives you the most freedom. You may feel that there are no classes that would work for you or no friend with whom to exercise. If so, start your own programme and review your needs and feelings periodically as you assess the success of your action plan.

A number of disease-specific voluntary organisations recommend exercise programmes. You can use their helpline numbers to find out about these. In some cases there are local branches meeting in local venues.

There is a wealth of tai chi, yoga, and other courses available in most communities. They are most often offered by your local adult education providers, but there are also many private tutors.

Most local authorities have leisure and recreation departments that run leisure centres. These include swimming pools, exercise suites, badminton, squash, and other indoor sports courts, where many specialist groups tend to meet. These are well worth exploring. There are always qualified instructors about who will talk to you about your personal needs even if you are starting from a very basic point. Their professional knowledge includes the needs of people with chronic conditions. By and large, classes and gyms are not expensive. In a few places, doctors can prescribe leisure centre courses.

Hospitals commonly offer medically-supervised exercise classes for people with heart or lung disease. Occasionally, people with other chronic illnesses can be included as well. These programmes are always free and have the advantage of medical supervision, if that's important to you.

Health and fitness clubs usually offer aerobic studios, weight training, cardiovascular equipment, and sometimes a heated pool. For all these services the fees can be high. The more luxurious the centre, the higher the price. Sometimes these facilities are available at quite reasonable prices to local people at four-star and five-star hotels. The key thing for a beginner to ask about is low-impact programmes, or classes for over-50s if this is appropriate. The qualifications of the staff can vary. Gather all the information you can and find the people and the place that feel right for you. These are some of the facilities to look for:

1. Classes designed for moderate and low-intensity exercise and for beginners. You should be able to observe classes and participate in at least one class before signing up and paying.

2. Instructors with qualifications and experience. Knowledgeable instructors are more likely to understand special needs and be willing and able to work with you.

3. Membership policies and fees that suit your diary and financial circumstances. They may allow you to pay only for a session of classes or let you "freeze" your membership at times when you can't participate. Some gyms offer different rates depending on how many services you use.

4. Facilities that are easy to get to, park near and enter. Dressing rooms and exercise sites should be accessible and safe, with professional staff on site.
5. A pool timetable that allows you to follow your programme. For example, some pools have times that are reserved for swimmers, rather than families, so that you can swim freely when the water isn't crowded. Some have women-only sessions.

6. Staff and other members whom you feel comfortable being around.

There are many excellent videotapes and DVDs for use at home. These vary in intensity, from very gentle chair exercises to more strenuous aerobic exercise. Ask your doctor, physiotherapist or disease-specific voluntary organisation for suggestions, or review the available material yourself.

Putting Your Programme Together

The best way to enjoy and keep up your exercise programme is to suit yourself! Choose what you want to do, a place where you feel comfortable, and an exercise time that fits your schedule. A woman who wants to have dinner on the table at 6 o'clock won't keep up an exercise programme that requires her to leave home for a 5 o'clock class. A retired man who enjoys lunch with friends and an afternoon nap is wise to choose an early- or mid-morning exercise time.

Pick two or three activities you think you would enjoy and that wouldn't put undue stress on your body. Choose activities that can be easily worked into your daily routine. If an activity is new to you, try it out before going to the expense of buying equipment or joining a health club. By having more than one exercise, you can keep active while adapting to holidays, seasons, and changing problems with your condition. Variety also helps keep you from getting bored.

Having fun and enjoying yourself are benefits of exercise that often go unmentioned. Too often we think of exercise as serious business. However, most people who stay with a programme do so because they enjoy it. They think of their exercise as recreation rather than a chore. Start off with success in mind, applying your visualisation techniques to "seeing" yourself doing the activity regularly and yourself feeling better afterwards. Allow yourself time to get used to new experiences and meet new people. You'll probably find that you look forward to exercise.

By making a conscious decision to get fitter, by applying action planning, by gathering proper information and by taking your first step, you will have taken control. When in the past you may have been told simply to "exercise more on your own," you will now have worked out the "how" and "when" for yourself. Having fully understood the benefits, you are more likely to keep going. Experience, practice and success help us establish a habit.

1. Keep your exercise goal in mind.
2. Choose exercises you want to do. Combine activities that move you towards your goal. Select exercises and activities from the next two chapters to get started.
3. Choose the time and place to exercise. Tell your family and friends about your plan.
4. Make an action plan with yourself. Decide how long you'll continue with these particular exercises. Six to eight weeks is a reasonable time commitment for a new programme.
5. Make an exercise journal or calendar on which you log the facts, whichever suits you. A journal will let you record more information. Choose what you like - the point is to have fun and enjoy being active.
6. Do some self-tests to keep track of your progress. You will find these at the end of the next two chapters. Record the date and results of the ones you choose. It can be a splendid boost to your motivation to compare the results of tests later on.
7. Start your programme. Begin gradually and proceed slowly, especially if you haven't exercised for a while.
8. Repeat the self-tests at regular intervals, record the results and check the changes.
9. Revise your programme. At the end of your six to eight weeks, decide what you liked, what worked and what made exercising difficult. Modify your programme and plan to go on for another few weeks. You may decide to change some exercises, the place or time you exercise, or your exercise partner.
10. Reward yourself for a job well done. Many people who start an exercise programme find that the rewards come with improved fit-

ness and endurance. Being able to enjoy family outings, a refreshing walk, or trips to the shops, the library, a concert or a museum are great rewards to look forward to.

Keeping It Up

If you haven't exercised recently, you'll undoubtedly experience some new sensations and even mild discomfort in the early days. It's normal to feel muscle tension and possible tenderness around joints, and to be a bit more tired in the evenings. Muscle or joint pain that lasts more than two hours after the exercise, or feeling tired into the next day, means that you have probably done too much too soon. Don't stop. Just exercise less vigorously or for a shorter amount of time the next day. When you do aerobic exercise, it's natural to feel your heart beat faster, your breathing speed up, and your body get warmer. However, feeling chest pain, excessive shortness of breath, nausea, or dizziness is not what you want. If this happens to you, stop exercising and discontinue your programme until you check with your doctor. (See Table 6.1.)

People who have a chronic illness often have additional sensations to sort out. It can be difficult at first to work out whether it is the illness or the exercise or both that is causing them. Talking to someone else who has had experience starting a new exercise programme can be a big help. Once you've sorted out the new sensations, you'll be able to exercise with confidence.

Realistically, expect setbacks. During the first year, people average two to three interruptions in their exercise schedule, often because of minor injuries or illnesses unrelated to their exercise. You may find yourself sidelined or derailed temporarily. Don't be discouraged. Try a different activity or simply rest. When you are feeling better, start again, but begin at a lower, gentler level. As a rule of thumb, it will take you the same amount of time to get back into shape as you were out. For instance, if you missed three weeks, it may take that long to get back to your previous level. Go slowly. Be kind to yourself. You can take the long-term view now you are committed.

Think of your head as the coach and your body as your team. For success, all parts of the team need attention. Be a good coach. Encourage and praise yourself. Design activities you feel your team can execute successfully. Choose places that are safe and hospitable. A good coach knows his or her team, sets good goals, and helps the team succeed. A good coach is loyal. A good coach does not belittle, nag, or make anyone feel guilty. Be a good coach to your team.

Table 7.1 *Advice for Exercise Problems*

Problem	Advice
Irregular or very rapid heartbeats	Stop exercising. Check your pulse. Are the beats regular or irregular? How fast is your heartbeat? Make a note of these and discuss this information with your doctor before exercising again. (See page 94)
Pain, tightness, or pressure in the chest, jaw, arms, neck, or back	Stop exercising. Talk to your doctor. Don't exercise until it has been cleared by your doctor.
Unusual, extreme shortness of breath, persisting 10 minutes after you exercise	Notify your doctor and get clearance before exercising again.
Light-headedness, dizziness, fainting, cold sweat, or confusion.	Lie down with your feet up, or sit down and put your head between your legs. If it happens more than once, check with your doctor before you exercise again.
Excessive tiredness after exercise, especially if you're still tired 24 hours after you exercise	Don't exercise so vigorously next time. If the excessive tiredness persists, check with your doctor. Talk to your doctor before you exercise again.

Besides a good coach, everyone needs an enthusiastic cheerleader or two. Of course, you can be your own cheerleader, but being both coach and cheerleader is a lot to do. Successful exercisers usually have at least one family member or close friend who actively supports their exercise habit. Your cheerleader can exercise with you, help you get other chores done, praise your accomplishments, or just consider your exercise time when making plans. Sometimes cheerleaders pop up by themselves, but don't be bashful about asking for a hand.

With exercise experience you develop a sense of control over yourself and your condition. You learn how to vary your activities to fit in with your day-to-day needs. You know when to do less and when to do more. You know that a change in symptoms or a period of inactivity is usually only temporary and doesn't have to be devastating. You know you have the tools to get back on track again.

Give your exercise plan a chance to succeed. Set reasonable goals, review your progress, solve your problems and reward yourself. Stay motivated. Your body will thank you!

• • •

Suggested Further Reading

Anderson, Bob. *Stretching*. Bolinas, CA: Shelter Publications Inc. 2000

Dagleish, Julia. *Health and Fitness Handbook*. London: Longman, 2001.

Hamler, Brad. *Exercises for Multiple Sclerosis: A Safe and Effective Program to Fight Fatigue, Build Strength, and Improve Balance* New York: Hatherleigh Press, 2004

Hawkins, Jerald, Hawkins, Sandra *Walking for Fun and Fitness*. Belmont, Cal.: Wadsworth, 2000.

O'Driscoll, Erin Rohan, *Exercises for Arthritis: 100 Exercises for Healthy Living: A Safe and Effective Way to Increase Strength, Improve Flexibility, Gain Energy, and Reduce Pain*. New York: Hatherleigh Press, 2007

Quotation at the top of the chapter is from J H Bland and S M Cooper,

CHAPTER 7

Exercising for Flexibility and Strength: Warm-Up and Cool-Down

You can use the exercises in this chapter in several ways. You can get in shape for more vigorous aerobic exercise, you can do something inside on days when you don't do aerobic exercise, and you can use them as part of your warm-up and cool-down routines. Choose exercises to build a strengthening and flexibility programme for the whole body. You can also choose specific exercises to improve your balance.

The exercises are arranged in order from the head and neck down to the toes. Most of the upper-body exercises may be done either sitting or standing. Exercises done lying down can be performed on the floor or on a firm mattress.

Exercises that are "Very Important for Posture" are labelled "VIP". Exercises to improve balance by strengthening and loosening legs and ankles are marked "BB"—Better Balance. There is also a final section of Balance Exercises designed to help you practise balance skills.

You might enjoy creating a routine of exercises that flow together. Arrange them so that you don't have to get up and down too often. Exercising to music you like can really help.

These helpful tips apply to all the exercises that follow:

- Move slowly and gently. Do not bounce or jerk.
- To loosen tight muscles and limber up stiff joints, stretch just until you feel tension, hold for five to ten seconds, and then relax.
- Don't push your body until it hurts. Stretching should feel pleasant, not painful.

- Start with no more than five repetitions of any exercise. Take at least two weeks to increase to ten repetitions.
- Always do the same number of exercises for your left side as for your right.
- Breathe naturally. Do not hold your breath. Count out loud to make sure you are breathing easily.
- If you feel increased symptoms that last more than two hours after exercising, next time do fewer repetitions, or eliminate an exercise that seems to be causing the symptoms. Don't abandon exercising.
- Change the exercises to suit you—ask a consultant if you're not sure if you're changing them too much. They are designed and illustrated to include both sides of the body and the full range of motion. If you're limited by muscle weakness or joint tightness, go ahead and do the exercise as completely as you can. The benefit of doing an exercise comes from moving towards a certain position, not from being able to complete the movement perfectly. In some cases you may find that after a while you can complete the movement. Otherwise, carry on with your own version.

Neck Exercises

1. Heads Up (VIP)

This exercise relieves jaw, neck, and upper back tension or pain, and is the start of good posture. You can do it while sitting at a desk, sewing, reading, or exercising. Just sit or stand straight and gently slide your chin back. Keep looking forward as your chin moves backward. You'll feel the back of your neck lengthen and straighten. To help, put your finger on your nose and then draw straight back from your finger. Don't worry about a little double chin—you really look much better with your neck straight!

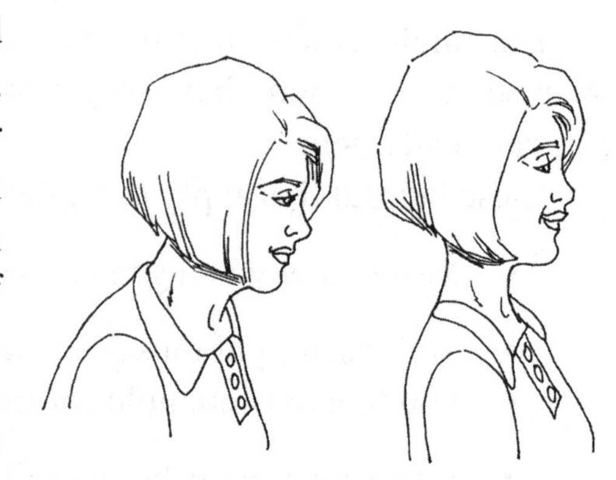

Clues for finding the correct position:

1. Ear over shoulder, not out in front
2. Head balanced over neck and trunk, not in the lead
3. Back of neck more vertical, not leaning forward
4. Bit of a double chin

2. Neck Stretch

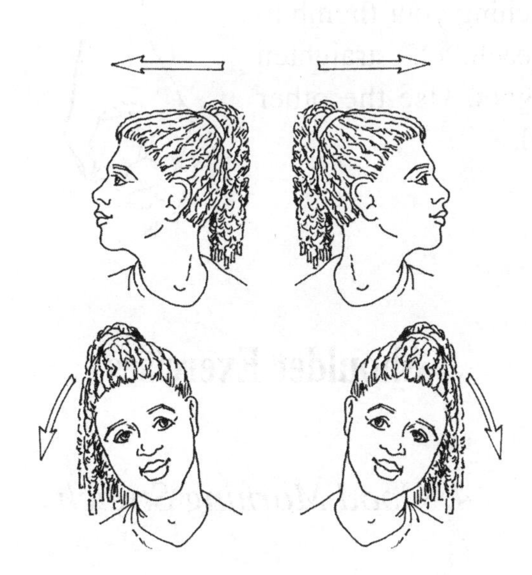

In heads-up position (Exercise 1) and with your shoulders relaxed:

1. Turn slowly to look over your right shoulder. Then turn slowly to look over your left shoulder.
2. Tilt your head to the right and then to the left. Move your ear toward your shoulder. Do not move your shoulder up to your ear.

Don't do these exercises if they cause neck pain, or pain or numbness in your arms or hands.

Hand and Wrist Exercises

A good place to do hand exercises is at a table that supports your forearms. Do them after washing dishes, after bathing, or when taking a break from working with your hands. Your hands are warmer and more supple at these times.

3. Thumb Walk

Holding your wrist straight, form the letter "O" by lightly touching your thumb to each fingertip. After each "O," straighten and spread your fingers. Use the other hand to help if needed.

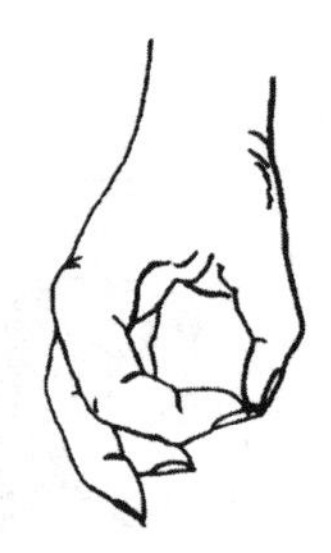

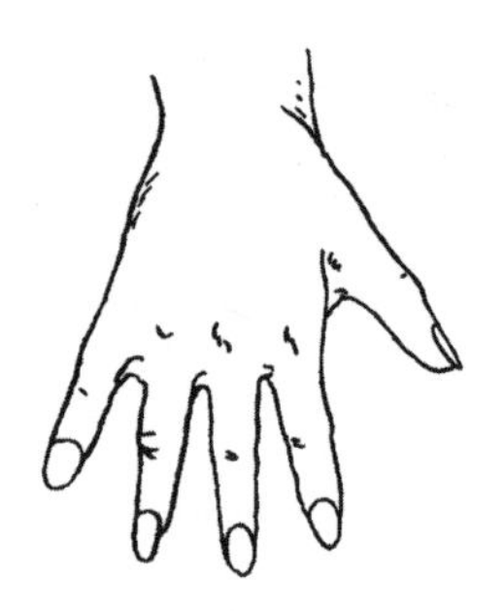

Shoulder Exercises

4. Good Morning Stretch

Start with hands in gentle fists, palms turned away from you, and wrists crossed. Breathe in and extend fingers while you uncross your arms and reach up as high as you can. Breathe out and relax.

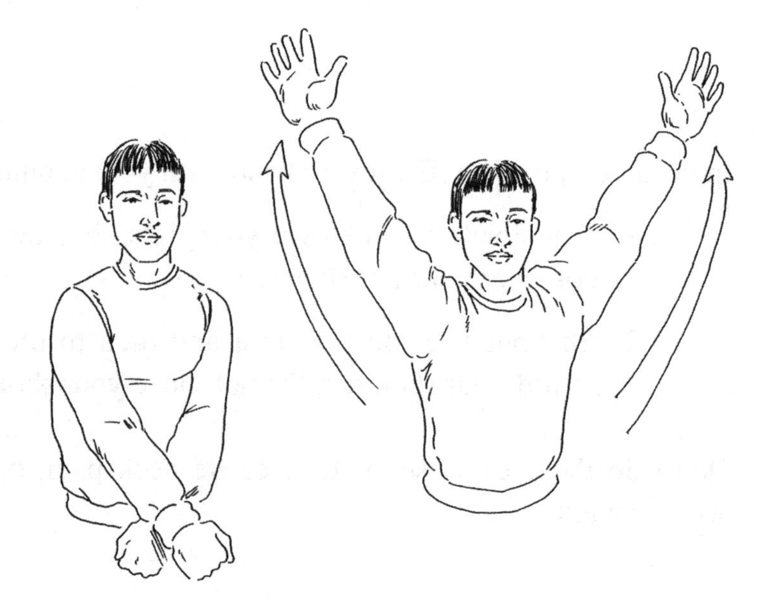

5. Broom Handle Exercise

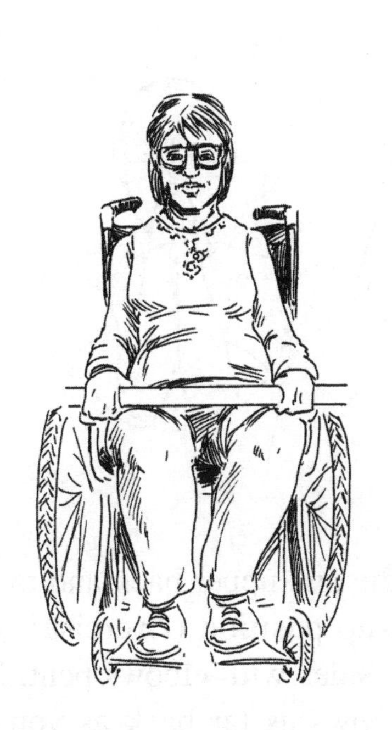

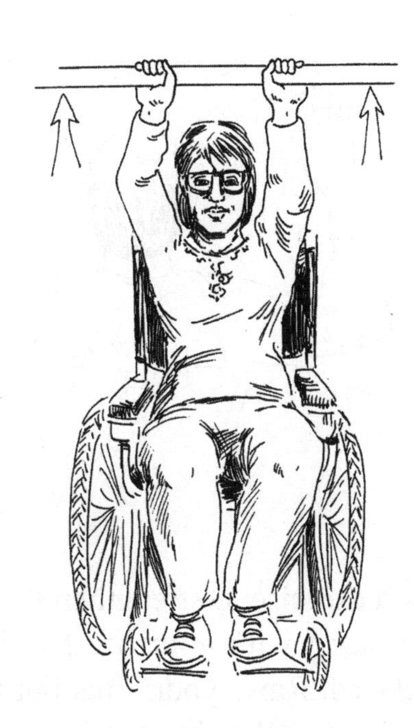

If one or both of your shoulders are tight or weak, you may want to give yourself a "helping hand." This shoulder exercise and the next allow the arms to help each other.

Use an actual broom or mop handle, a walking stick, or a strong garden cane. Place one hand on each end and raise the stick as high overhead as possible. You might try this in front of the mirror. This exercise can be done standing, sitting, or lying down.

6. Pat and Reach

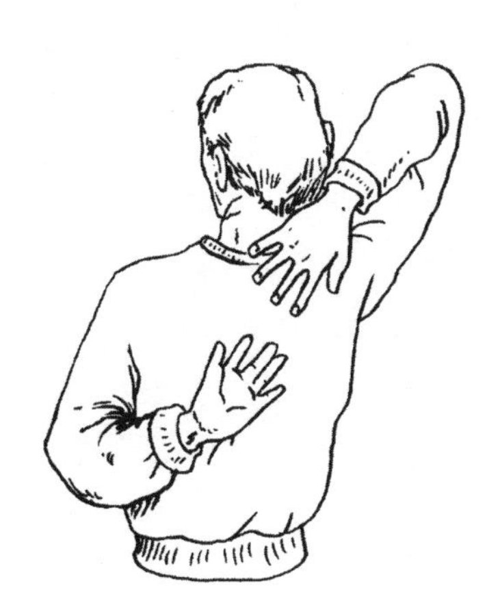

This double-duty exercise helps increase flexibility and strength for both shoulders. Raise one arm up over your head, and bend your elbow to pat yourself on the back. Move your other arm to your back, bend your elbow, and reach up toward the other hand. Can your fingertips touch? Relax and switch arm positions. Can you touch on that side? For most people, one side is easier than the other.

7. Shoulder Blade Pinch (VIP)

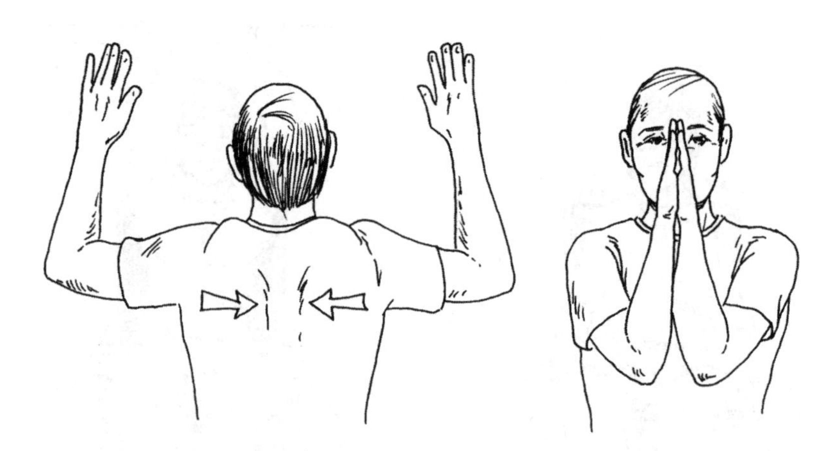

This is a good exercise to strengthen the middle and upper back and to stretch the chest. Sit or stand with your head in heads-up position (Exercise 1) and your shoulders relaxed. Raise your arms out to the sides with elbows bent. Pinch your shoulder blades together by moving your elbows as far back as you can. Hold briefly, then slowly move your arms forward to touch elbows. If this position is uncomfortable, lower your arms or rest your hands on your shoulders.

Back and Abdominal Exercises

8. *Knee to Chest Stretch*

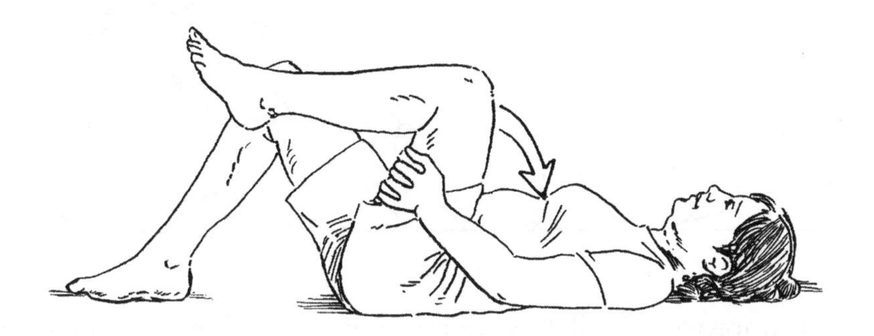

For a low back stretch, lie on the floor with knees bent and feet flat. Bring one knee toward your chest, using your hands to help. Hold your knee near your chest for ten seconds and lower the leg slowly. Repeat with the other knee. You can also tuck both legs at the same time if you wish. Relax and enjoy the stretch.

9. *Pelvic Tilt (VIP)*

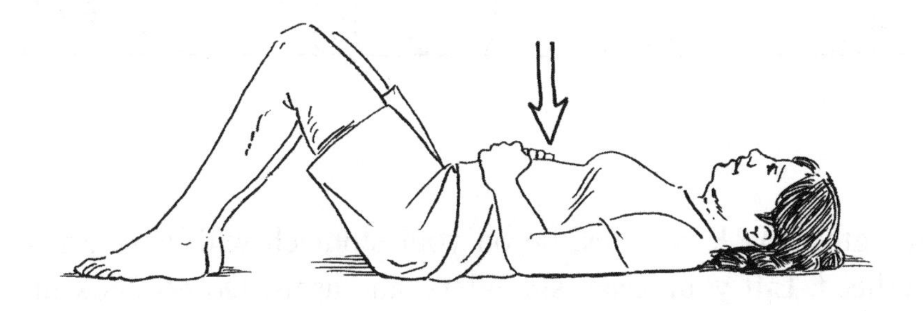

This is an excellent exercise for the low back. Lie on your back with knees bent, feet flat. Place your hands on your abdomen. Flatten the small of your back against the floor by tightening your stomach muscles and your buttocks. It helps to imagine bringing your pubic bone to your chin, or trying to pull your tummy in enough to zip up a tight pair of trousers. Hold the tilt for five to ten seconds. Relax. Arch your back slightly. Relax and repeat the Pelvic Tilt. Keep breathing. Count the seconds out loud. Once you've mastered the Pelvic Tilt lying down, practise it sitting, standing, and walking.

10. Back Lift (VIP)

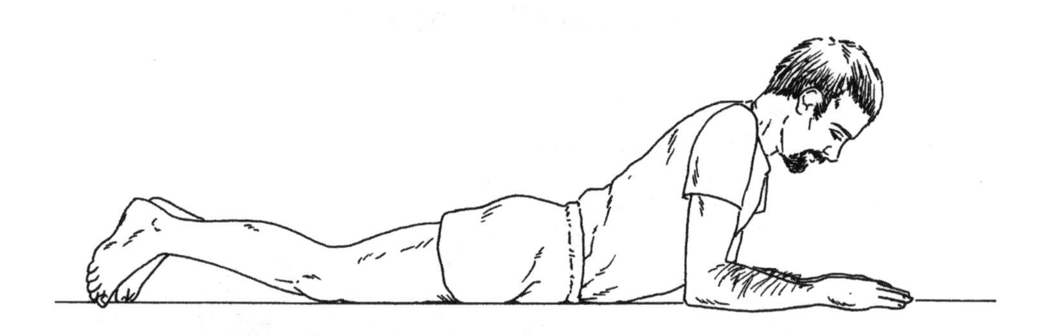

1. This exercise improves flexibility along your spine. Lie on your stomach and rise up onto your forearms. Keep your back relaxed, and keep your stomach and hips down. If this is comfortable, straighten your elbows. Breathe naturally and relax for at least ten seconds. If you have moderate to severe low back pain, do not do this exercise unless it has been specifically prescribed for you.

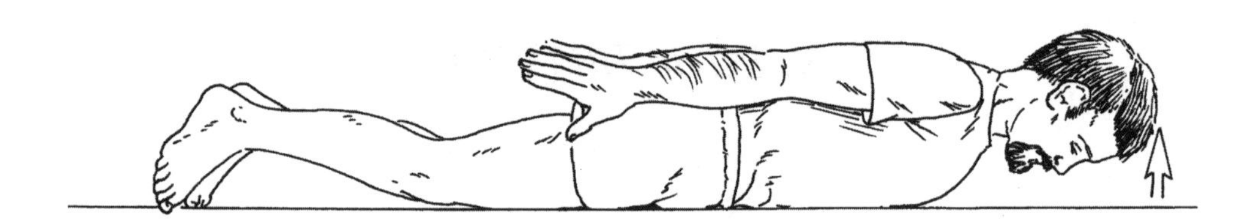

2. To strengthen back muscles, lie on your stomach with your arms at your side or overhead. Lift your head, shoulders, and arms. Do not look up. Keep looking down with your chin tucked in. Count out loud as you hold for a count of 10. Relax. You can also lift your legs, instead of your head and shoulders, off the floor.

Lifting both ends of your body at once is a fairly strenuous exercise. It may not be helpful for a person with back pain.

11. Low Back Rock and Roll

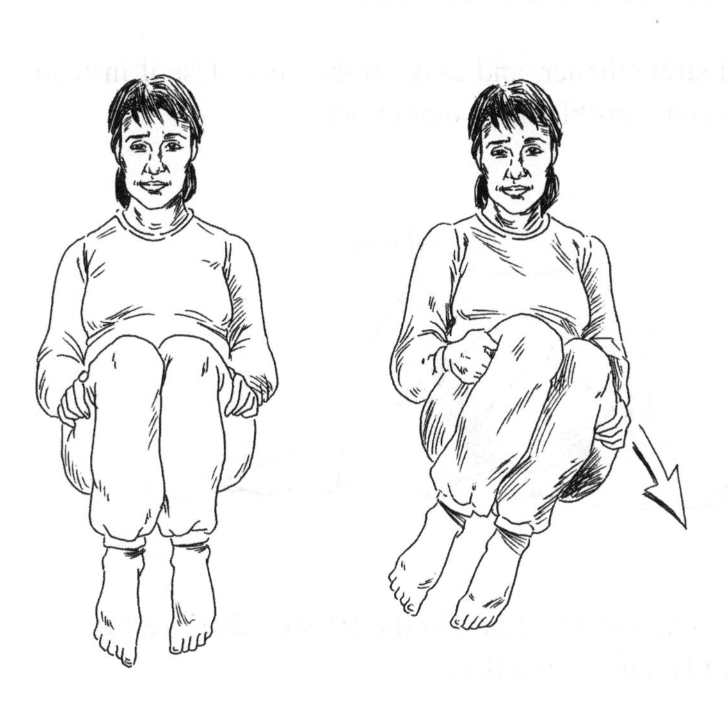

Lie on your back and pull your knees up to your chest with your hands behind the thighs. Rest in this position for ten seconds, then gently roll knees from one side to the other, rocking your hips back and forth. Keep your upper back and shoulders flat on the ground.

12. Curl-Up

A curl-up, as shown here, is a good way to strengthen abdominal muscles. Lie on your back, knees bent, feet flat. Do the Pelvic Tilt (Exercise 9). Slowly curl up to raise your head and shoulders. Uncurl back down, or hold for ten seconds and slowly lower. Breathe out as you curl up, and breathe in as you go back down. Don't hold your breath. If you have neck problems, or if your neck hurts when you do this exercise, try the next one instead. Never tuck your feet under a chair or have someone hold your feet!

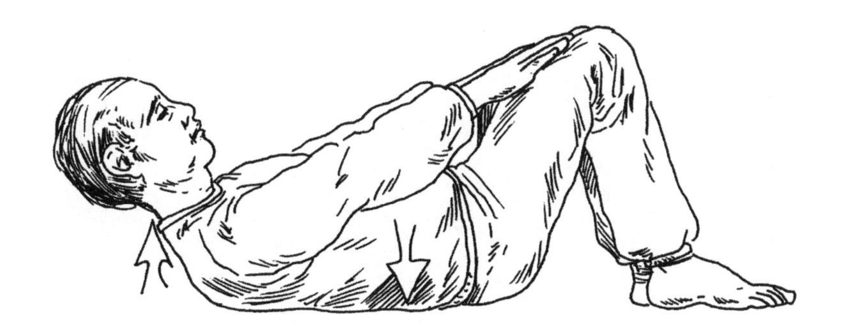

13. Roll-Out

This is another good abdominal strengthener, and easy on the neck. Use it instead of the curl-up, or, if neck pain is not a problem, do them both.

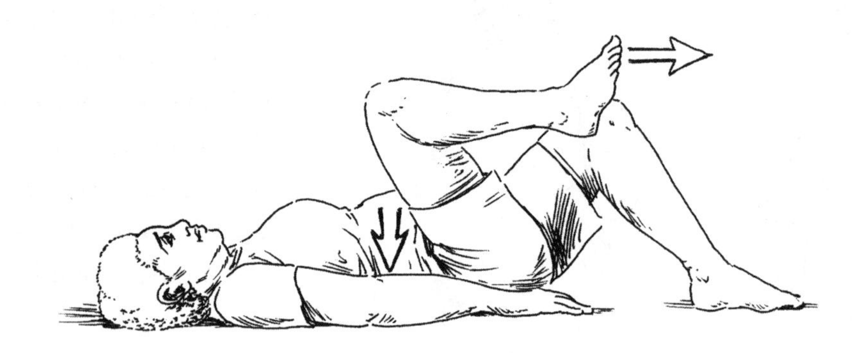

1. Lie on your back with knees bent and feet flat. Do the Pelvic Tilt (Exercise 9), and hold your lower back firmly against the floor.

2. Slowly and carefully, move one leg away from your chest as you straighten your knee. Move your leg out until you feel your lower back start to arch. When this happens, tuck your knee back to your chest. Reset your pelvic tilt and roll your leg out again. Breathe out as your leg rolls out. Do not hold your breath. Repeat with the other leg.

You are strengthening your abdominal muscles by holding your pelvic tilt against the weight of your leg. As you get stronger, you'll be able to straighten your legs out farther and move both legs together.

Hip and Leg Exercises

14. Straight Leg Raises

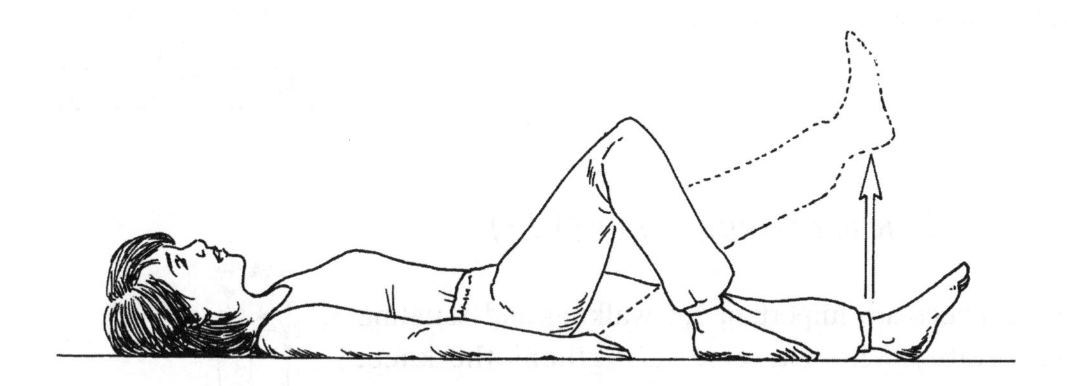

This exercise strengthens the muscles that bend the hip and straighten the knee. Lie on your back, knees bent, feet flat. Straighten one leg. Tighten the muscle on the top of that thigh, and straighten the knee as much as possible. Keeping the knee straight, raise your leg one to two feet (about 50 cm) off the ground. Do not arch your back. Hold your leg up and count out loud for ten seconds. Relax. Repeat with the other leg.

15. Hip Hooray

This exercise can be done standing or lying on your back. If you lie down, spread your legs as far apart as possible. Roll your legs and feet out like a duck, then in to be pigeon-toed, move your legs back together. If you are standing, move one leg out to your side as far as you can. Lead out with the heel and in with the toes. Hold on to a worktop for support.

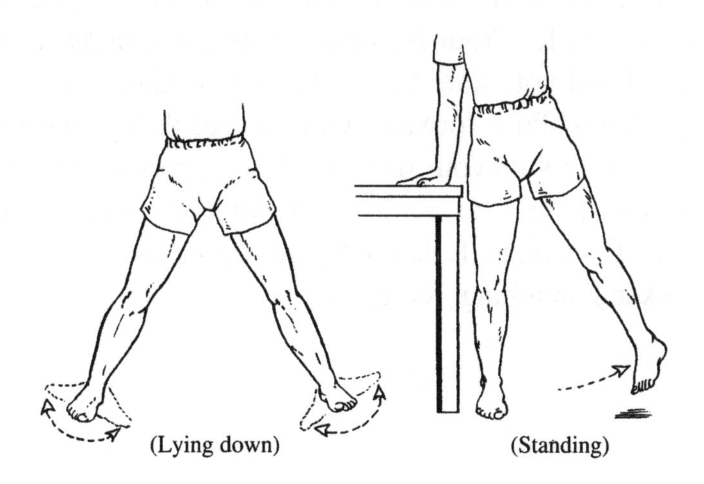

16. Back Kick (VIP)

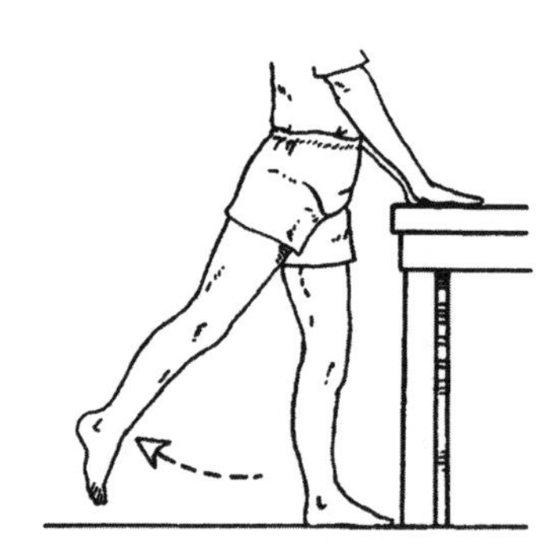

This exercise increases the backward mobility and strength of your hip. Hold on to a worktop for support. Move the leg up and back, knee straight. Stand up straight, and do not lean forward.

17. Knee Strengthener (VIP)

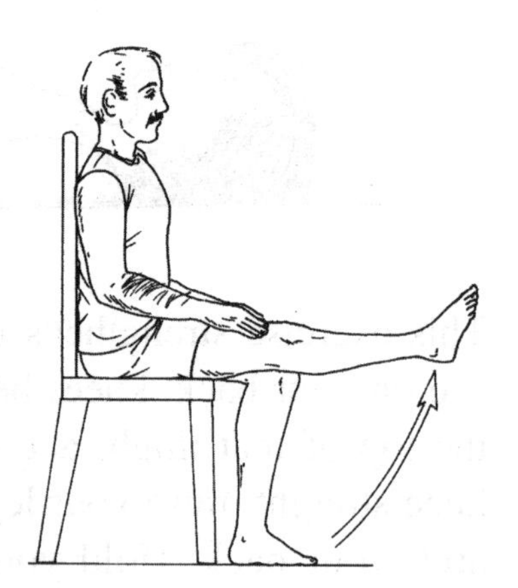

Strong knees are important for walking and standing comfortably. This exercise strengthens the knee. Sitting in a chair, straighten the knee by tightening up the muscle on top of your thigh. Place your hand on your thigh and feel the muscle work. If you wish, make circles with your toes. As your knee strengthens, see if you can build up to holding your leg out for 30 seconds. Count out loud. Do not hold your breath.

18. Power Knees

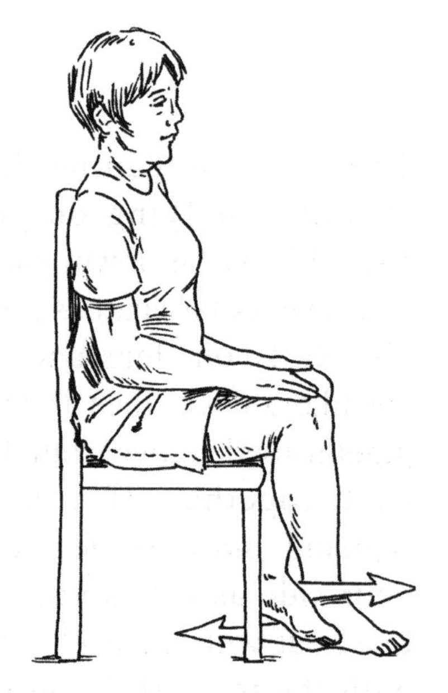

This exercise strengthens the muscles that bend and straighten your knee. Sit in a chair and cross your legs at the ankles. Your legs can be almost straight, or you can bend your knees as much as you like. Try several positions. Push forward with your back leg, and press backward with your front leg. Exert pressure evenly so that your legs do not move. Hold and count out loud for 10 seconds. Relax. Change leg positions. Be sure to keep breathing. Repeat.

19. Ready-Go (VIP) (BB)

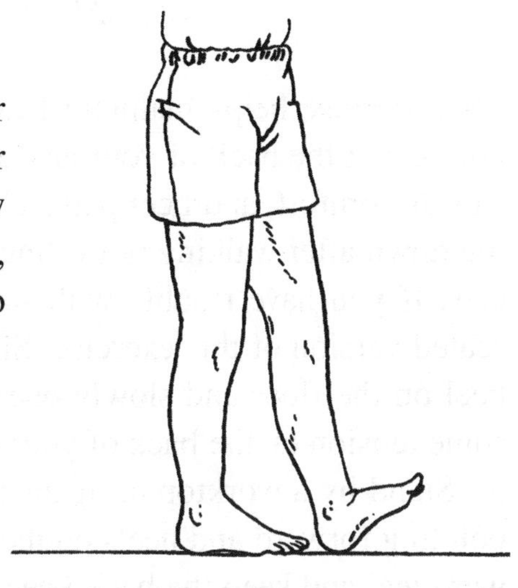

Stand with one leg slightly in front of the other in the position of having your heel on the floor ready to take a step with the front foot. Now tighten the muscles on the front of your thigh, making your knee firm and straight. Hold to count of 10. Relax. Repeat with the other leg.

20. Hamstring Stretch

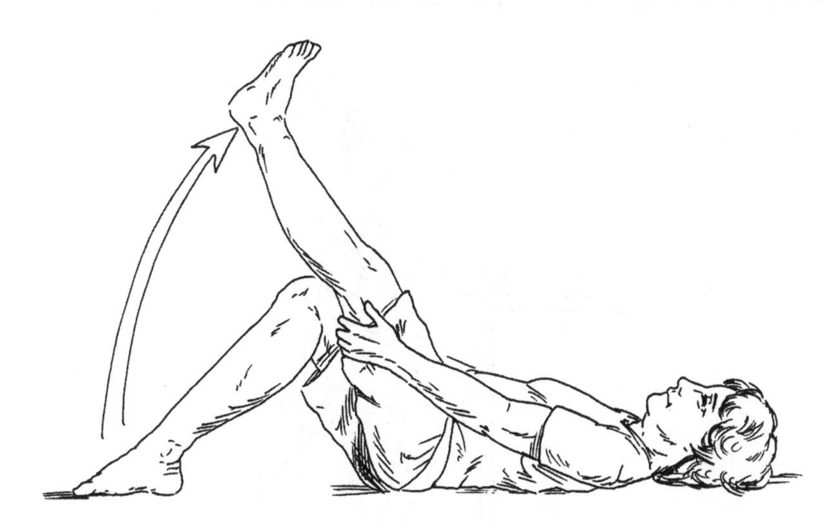

Do the self-test for hamstring tightness (page 88) to see if you need to do this exercise. If you have unstable knees, or "back knee"—a knee that curves backward when you stand up—do not do this exercise.

If you do have tight hamstrings, lie on your back, knees bent, feet flat. Grasp one leg at a time behind the thigh. Holding the leg out at arm's length, slowly straighten the knee. Hold the leg as straight as you can as you count to 10. You should feel a slight stretch at the back of your knee and thigh.

Be careful with this exercise. It's easy to overstretch and cause discomfort.

21. Achilles Stretch (BB)

This exercise helps maintain flexibility in the Achilles tendon, the large tendon you feel at the back of your ankle. Good flexibility helps reduce the risk of injury, calf discomfort, and heel pain. The Achilles Stretch is especially helpful for cooling down after walking or cycling, and for people who get cramps in the calf muscles. If you have trouble with standing balance or muscle spasms, you can do a seated version of this exercise. Sit in a chair with feet flat on the floor. Keep your heel on the floor and slowly one foot at a time back to bend your ankle and feel some tension on the back of your calf.

Stand by a worktop or against a wall. Place one foot in front of the other, toes pointing forward and heels on the ground. Lean forward, bend the knee of the forward leg, and keep the back knee straight, heel down. You will feel a good stretch in the calf. Hold the stretch for ten seconds. Do not bounce. Move gently.

It's easy to get sore round your heel doing this exercise. If you've worn shoes with high heels for a long time, be particularly careful.

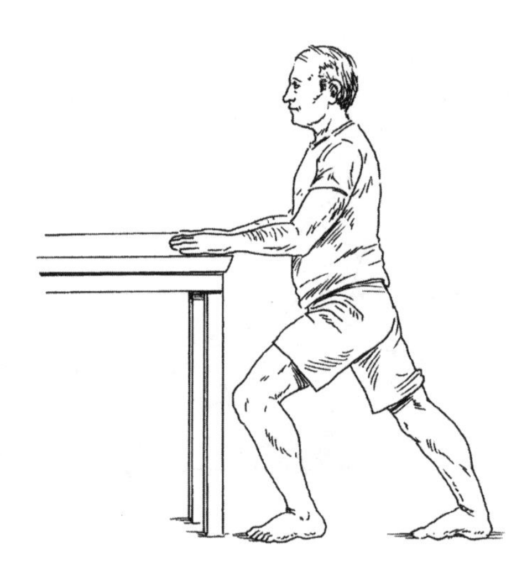

22. Tiptoes (BB)

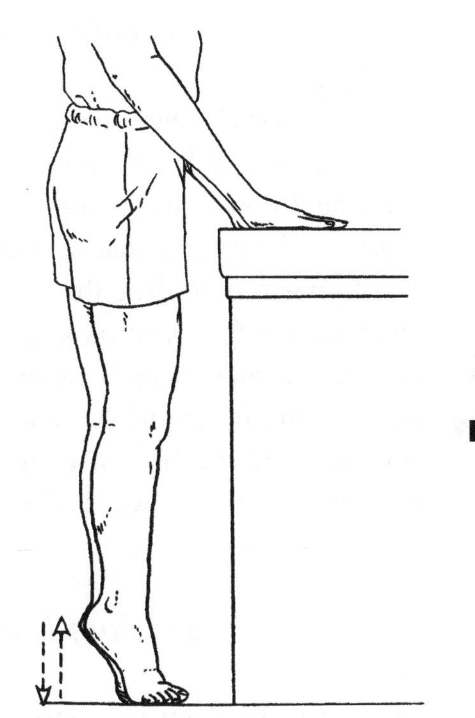

This exercise will help strengthen your calf muscles and make walking, climbing stairs, and standing less tiring. It may also improve your balance. Hold on to a worktop or table for support and stand on your tiptoes. Hold for ten seconds. Lower slowly. How high you go is not as important as keeping your balance and controlling your ankles. It is easier to do both legs at the same time. If your feet are too sore to do this standing, start doing it while sitting down. If this exercise makes your ankle jerk, leave it out, and talk to your physiotherapist about other ways to strengthen these calf muscles if needed.

Ankle and Food Exercises

Do these exercises sitting in a straight-backed chair with your feet bare. Have a bath towel and ten marbles next to you. These exercises are for flexibility, strength, and comfort. This is a good time to examine your feet and toes for any signs of circulation or skin problems, and check your nails to see if they need trimming.

23. Towel Grabber

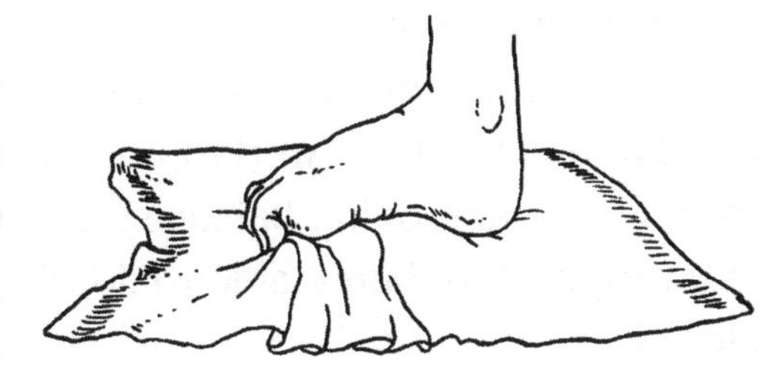

Spread a towel out in front of your chair. Place your feet on the towel, with your heels near the edge closest to you. Keep your heels down and your foot slightly raised. Scoot the towel back underneath your feet, by pulling it with your toes. When you have done as much as you can, reverse the toe motion and scoot the towel out again.

24. Marble Pick-Up

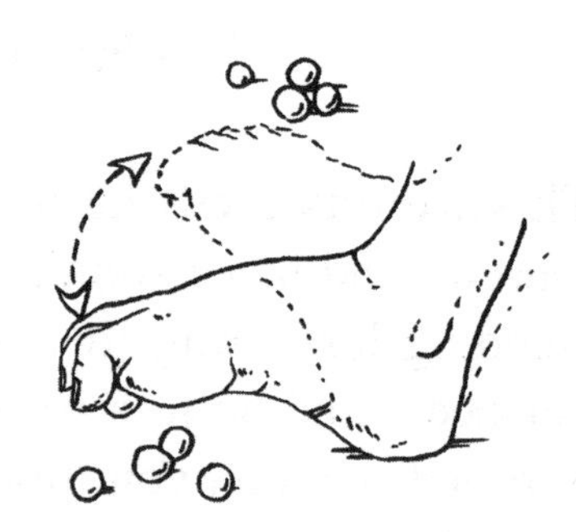

Do this exercise one foot at a time. Place several marbles on the floor between your feet. Keep your heel down, and pivot your toes toward the marbles. Pick up a marble with your toes, and pivot your foot to drop the marble as far as possible from where you picked it up. Repeat until all the marbles have been moved. Reverse the process and return all the marbles to the starting position. If marbles are difficult, try other objects, like dice or wads of paper.

25. Foot Roll

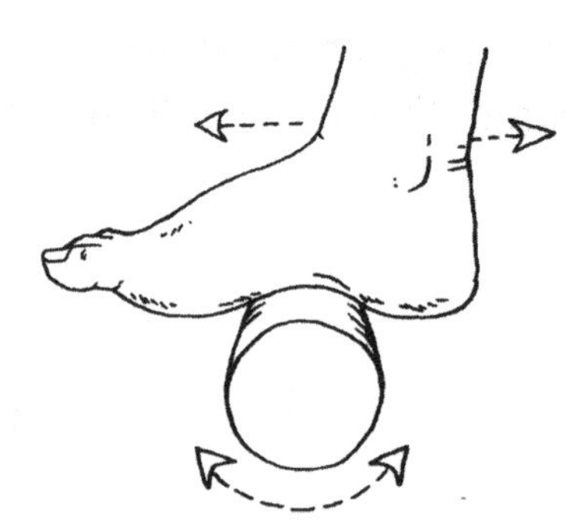

Place a rolling pin or a large dowel under the arch of your foot, and roll it back and forth. It feels very pleasant and stretches the ligaments in the arch of the foot.

Balance Exercises

The exercises in this section are designed to let you practise balance activities in a safe and progressive way. The exercises are presented in order of difficulty, so start with the first exercises and work up to the more difficult ones as your strength and balance improve. If you feel that your balance is particularly poor, exercise with someone else close by to give you a supporting hand if needed. Always practise by a worktop or stable chair so that you can hold on if you need to. Signs of improving balance are being able to hold a position longer or without extra support, or being able to do the exercise or hold the position with your eyes closed.

26. Beginning Balance

Stand quietly with your feet comfortably apart. Place your hands on your hips and turn your head and trunk as far to the left as possible, and then to the right. Repeat five to ten times. To increase the difficulty, close your eyes and do the same thing.

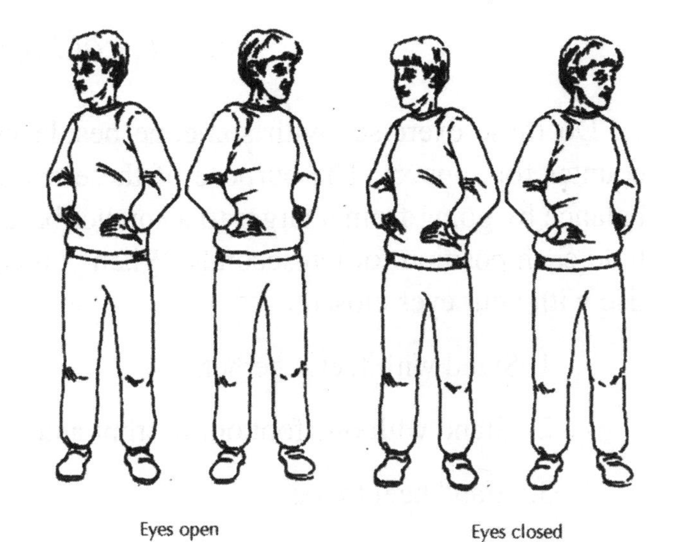

27. Swing and Sway

Using a worktop or the back of a stable chair for support, do each of the following five to ten times:

1. Rock back on your heels and then go up on your toes.
2. Do the box step, like dancing the waltz.
3. March in place with eyes open and eyes closed.

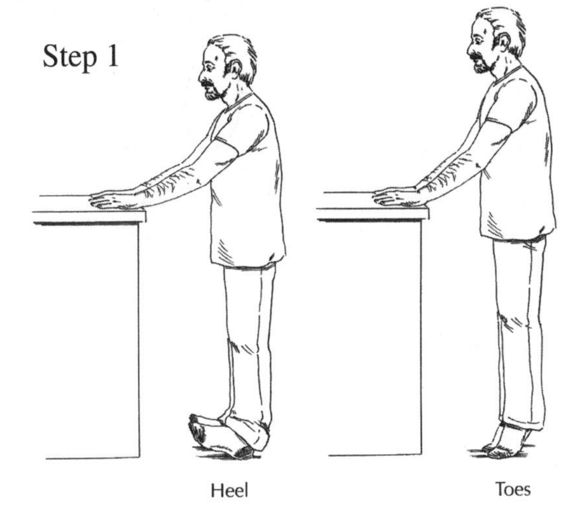

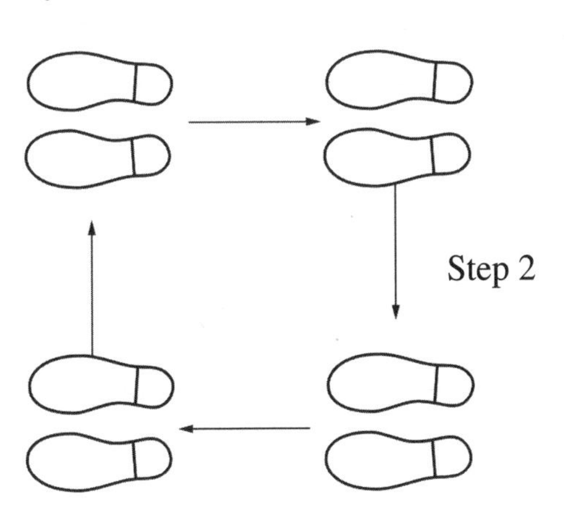

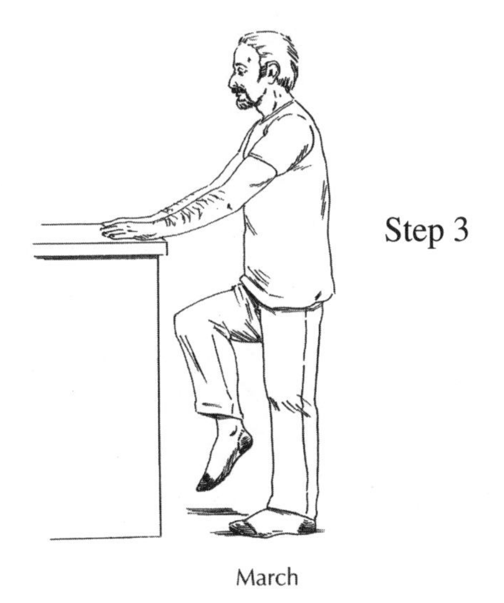

28. Base of Support

Do these exercises with someone beside you to help or standing close to a counter for support. The purpose of these exercises is to help you improve your balance by going from a larger to a smaller base of support. Work on being able to hold each position for ten seconds. When you can do it with your eyes open, practise with your eyes closed.

1. Stand with feet together.
2. Stand with one foot out in front and the other back.
3. Stand heel to toe.

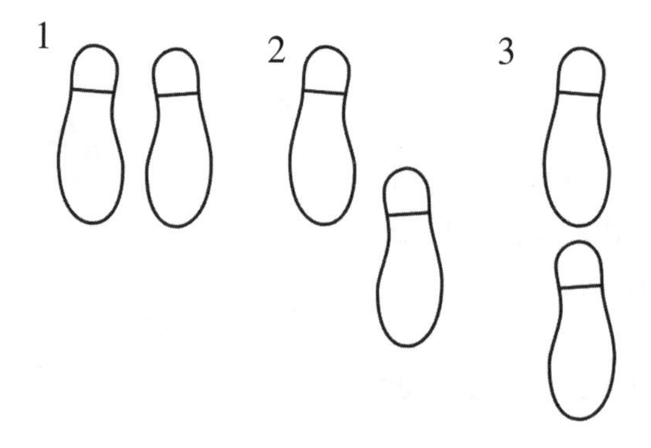

29. Toe Walk

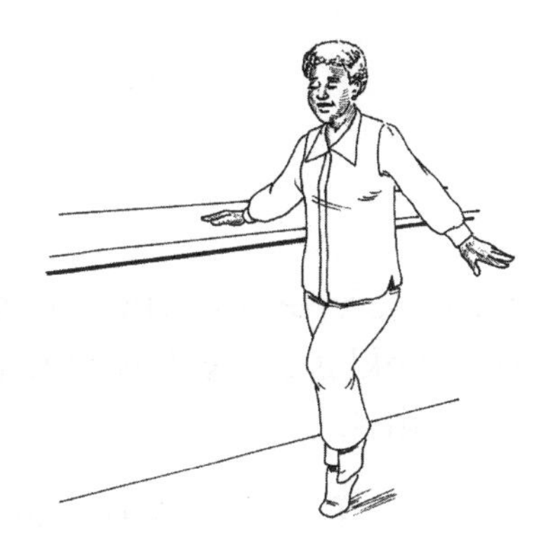

The purpose of this exercise is to increase ankle strength and to give you practice balancing on a small base of support while moving. Stay close to a worktop or other firm support. Rise up on your toes and walk up and back along the counter. Once you are comfortable walking on your toes without support and with your eyes open, try with your eyes closed.

30. Heel Walk

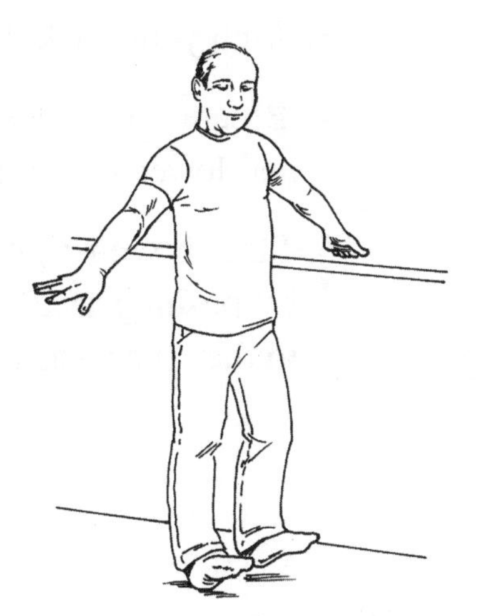

The purpose of this exercise is to increase your lower leg strength and give you practice moving on a small base of support. Stay close to a counter for support. Raise your toes and forefoot and walk up and back along the counter on your heels. Once you are comfortable walking on your heels without support and with your eyes open, try with your eyes closed.

31. One-Legged Stand

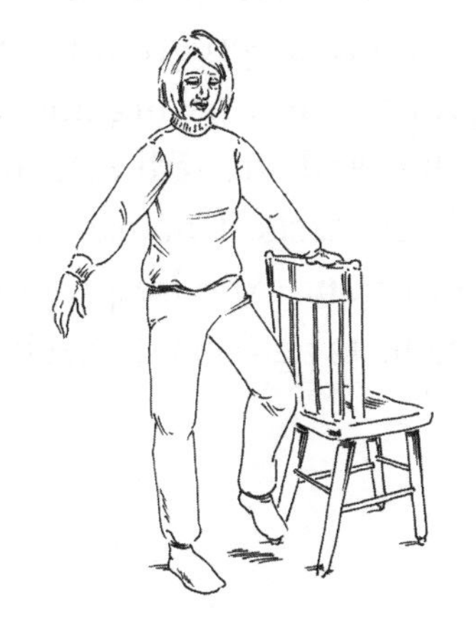

Holding onto a worktop or stable chair, lift one foot completely off the ground. Once you are balanced, lift your hand. The goal is to hold the position for ten seconds. Once you can do this for ten seconds without holding on, practise it with your eyes closed. Repeat with the other leg.

The Whole Body

32. The Stretcher

This exercise is a whole-body stretch to do lying on your back. Start the motion at your ankles as explained here, or reverse the process if you want to start with your arms first.

1. Point your toes, and then pull your toes toward your nose. Relax.
2. Bend your knees. Then flatten your knees and let them relax.
3. Arch your back. Do the Pelvic Tilt. Relax.
4. Breathe in, and stretch your arms above your head. Breathe out, and lower your arms. Relax.
5. Stretch your right arm above your head, and stretch your left leg by pushing away with your heel. Hold for a count of ten. Switch to the other side and repeat.

Self-Tests

Whatever our goals, we all need to see that our efforts make a difference. Since an exercise programme produces gradual change, it's often hard to tell if the programme is working and to recognise improvement. Choose several of these flexibility and strength tests to measure your progress. Not everyone will be able to do all the tests. Choose those that work best for you. Perform each test before you start your exercise programme, and record the results. After every four weeks, do the tests again and check your improvement.

1. Arm Flexibility

Do Exercise 6 (Pat and Reach) for both sides of the body. Ask someone to measure the distance between your fingertips

Goal: Less distance between your fingertips.

2. Shoulder Flexibility

Stand facing a wall, with your toes touching the wall. One arm at a time, reach up the wall in front of you. Hold a pencil, or have someone mark how far you reached. Also do this sideways, standing about three inches (8 cm) away from the wall.

Goal: To reach higher.

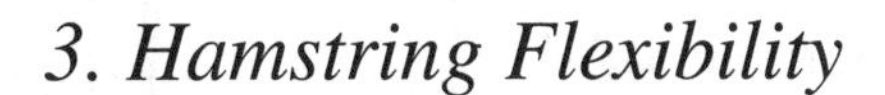

3. Hamstring Flexibility

Do the Hamstring Stretch (Exercise 20), one leg at a time. Keep your thigh perpendicular to your body. How much does your knee bend? How tight does the back of your leg feel?

Goal: Straighter knee and less tension in the back of the leg.

4. Ankle Flexibility

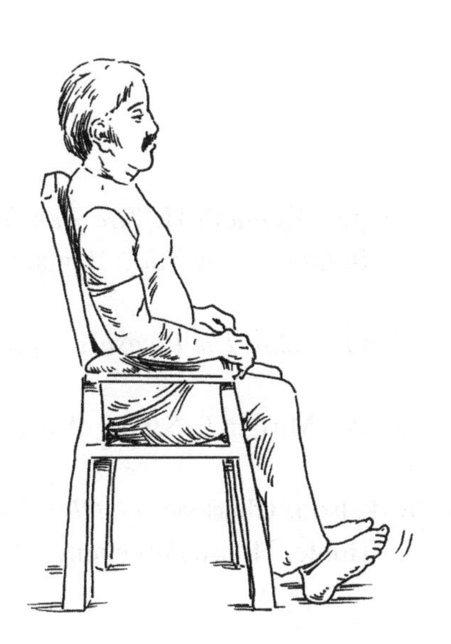

Sit in a chair with your bare feet flat on the floor and your knees bent at a 90- degree angle. Keep your heels on the floor. Raise your toes and the front of your foot. Ask someone to measure the distance between the ball of your foot and the floor.

Goal: One to two inches (3 to 5 cm) between your foot and the floor.

5. Abdominal Strength

Use the Curl-Up (Exercise 12). Count how many repetitions you can do before you get too tired to do more, or count how many you can do in one minute.

Goal: More repetitions.

6. Ankle Strength

This test has two parts.

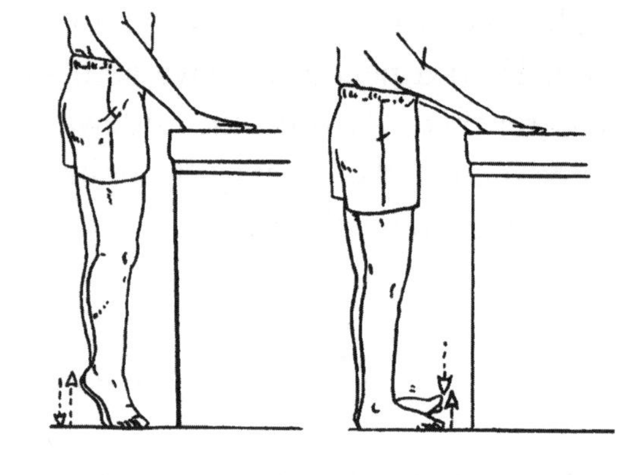

1. Stand at a table or worktop for support. Do Exercise 22 (Tiptoes) as quickly and as often as you can. How many can you do before you tire?

2. Stand with your feet flat. Put most of your weight on one foot, and quickly tap the floor with the front part of your other foot. How many taps can you do before you tire?

Goal: Ten to fifteen repetitions of each movement.

• • •

Suggested Further Reading

Cooper, Kenneth H. *The Aerobics Program for Total Well-Being: Exercise, Diet, Emotional Balance.* New York: Bantam Doubleday, 1985.

Jerome, John. *The Pleasures of Staying Supple.* London: Souvenir Press, 2000.

Nelson, Miriam E. *Strong Women Stay Young.* New York: Bantam Books, 1998.

Torkelson, Charlene. *Get Fit While You Sit: Easy Workout From Your Chair.* Berkeley, Calif.: Hunter House Publishing, 1999.

CHAPTER
8

Exercising for Endurance: Aerobic Activities

Gain without pain – smiles not miles

How much is enough? You've got to do enough to increase your endurance – but not so much you make yourself hurt! Action plans are invaluable for working out what's enough. Think through what your goals are, work out a detailed action plan, review it and revise it and don't forget the reward for a job well done.

The aerobic exercise we do to increase endurance is easy to *over*-do, even for those who don't have a chronic illness. Contrary to what you might have heard, you don't have to work very hard for exercise to do some good. Exhaustion, sore muscles, painful joints, and shortness of breath are the results of doing too much too soon. So don't be one of those people who give up, thinking that exercise is just not meant for them, just because they've gone at it too hard.

There's no exact measure of how much exercise you need. But some is definitely better than none. If you start slowly and increase gradually, you're likely to keep it up for life. It's generally better to underdo it at the start.

Several studies suggest that the upper limit of benefit is about two hundred minutes of moderate-intensity aerobic exercise per week—have look at the talk test below for what moderate intensity activity feels like. Doing more than that doesn't gain you much and it increases your risk of injury. On the other hand, doing one hundred minutes of exercise per week gets you about 90% of the gain, while sixty minutes of aerobic exercise per week yields about 75% of the gain. Sixty minutes equals fifteen minutes of mild aerobic exercise just four times a week!

How often? How long? How much? Use your consultants to sort out any specific answers which apply to your condition.

- **Frequency:** Five days a week is a good goal for aerobic exercise. Begin by taking every other day off to give your body a chance to rest and recover. It's a good idea anyway to rest at least one day a week.
- **Time:** Start with a few minutes, and gradually increase about thirty minutes a session. Once you get there, you can gradually increase the intensity. You could alternate intervals of brisk exercise with intervals of rest or easy exercise. For example, after three to five minutes of brisk walking, do one to two minutes of easy strolling, then another three to five minutes of brisk walking. When you're up to thirty minutes, gradually cut down the rest intervals until you can keep going for twenty to thirty minutes of brisk exercise. Or consider two sessions of ten to fifteen minutes each. Either way appears to improve health significantly.
- **Intensity:** Safe and effective endurance exercise should be done at no more than moderate intensity. Exercise intensity is measured by how hard you work. For a trained runner, completing a mile in twelve minutes is probably low-intensity exercise. For a person who hasn't exercised in a long time, a brisk ten-minute walk may be of moderate to high intensity. For others with severe physical limitations, one minute may be of moderate intensity. Work out what is moderate intensity for you. There are several easy ways to do this. Choose one which suits your particular situation and condition, and takes into account your medication.

Talk Test

Talk to another person or yourself, sing, or recite poems out loud while you exercise. Moderate-intensity exercise allows you to speak comfortably. If you can't carry on a conversation or sing because you are breathing too hard or are short of breath, you're working too hard. Slow down. The talk test is an easy way to regulate exercise intensity.

Perceived Exertion

Another way to monitor intensity is to rate how hard you're working on a scale of 0 to 10. Zero, at the low end of the scale, is lying down, doing no work at all. Ten is equivalent to working as hard as possible, very hard work that you couldn't do longer than a few seconds. Of course, you never want to exercise as hard as that. A good level for your aerobic exercise routine is between 3 and 6 on this scale. At this level, you'll usually feel warmer, that you're breathing more deeply and faster than usual, that your heart is beating faster than normal, but you should not be feeling pain.

Of course, these are just rough guidelines on frequency, duration, and intensity, not a rigid prescription. Listen to your own body. Sometimes you need to tell yourself, and maybe others, that enough is enough. More is not necessarily better.

Heart Rate

One way to measure the intensity of your exercise is to monitor your heart rate. The faster the heart beats, the harder you're working. Your heart also beats fast when you are frightened or nervous, but this is about how your heart responds to physical activity. Endurance exercise at moderate intensity raises your heart rate into a range between 60% and 80 % of your safe maximum heart rate. Your safe exercise heart rate gets lower as you get older. You can follow the general guidelines of, "Age–Exercise Heart Rate," or calculate your individual exercise heart rate. Either way, you need to know how to take your pulse.

Take your pulse by placing the tips of your middle three fingers at your wrist below the base of your thumb. Feel around in that spot until you feel the pulsations of blood pumping with each heartbeat. Count how many beats you feel in fifteen seconds. Multiply this number by 4 to find out how fast your heart is beating in one minute. Start by taking your pulse whenever you think of it, and you'll soon learn the difference between your resting and exercise heart rates.

The exercise heart rate range in our example is from 96 to 128 beats per minute. What is yours?

Most people count their pulse for fifteen seconds, not a whole minute. To find your 15-second pulse, divide both the lower-end and upper-end numbers by 4. The person in our example should be able to count between 24 (96 ÷ 4) and 32 (128 ÷ 4) beats in 15 seconds while exercising.

How to Calculate Your Own Exercise Heart Rate Range

1. Subtract your age from 220:
   Example: 220 – 60 = 160 You: 220 – ______ = ______
2. To find the lower end of your exercise heart rate range, multiply your answer in step 1 by [.6]:
   Example: 160 × .6 = 96 You: ______ × .6 = ______
3. To find the upper end of your exercise heart rate range, which you should not exceed, multiply your answer in step 1 by [.8]:
   Example: 160 × .8 = 128 You: ______ × .8 = ______

The most important reason for knowing your exercise heart rate range is so that you can learn not to exercise too vigorously. After you've done your warm-up and five minutes of endurance exercise, take your pulse. If it's higher than the upper rate, don't panic. Slow down a bit. Don't work so hard.

At first, some people have trouble keeping their heart rate within the "ideal" heart rate range. Don't worry about that. Keep exercising at the level with which you're most comfortable. As you get more experienced and stronger, you will gradually be able to do more vigorous exercise while keeping your heart rate within your "goal" range. But don't let the target heart rate monitoring become a burden. Even low-intensity exercise can benefit you significantly. So use the "ideal" heart rate range as a rough guide, but don't worry if you can't reach the lower end of that range. Just keep exercising!

If you are taking medicine that regulates your heart rate, have trouble feeling your pulse, or think that keeping track of your heart rate is a bother, use one of the other methods to monitor your exercise intensity.

The FIT Formula—How much IS enough!

The results of your aerobic exercise programme depend on how often you exercise (F = Frequency), how hard you work (I = Intensity), and how long you exercise each day (T = Time). In much the same way a doctor prescribes medicine to have a certain effect, you can select your own "exercise dose" to get the result

Table 8.1 *Age–Exercise Heart Rate*

Age Range	Exercise Pulse (15 sec)	Exercise Pulse (1 min)
0–30	29–39	116–156
30–40	28–37	112–148
40–50	26–35	104–140
50–60	25–33	100–132
60–70	23–31	92–124
70–80	22–29	88–116
80+	16–24	64–96

you want. Your exercise dose comes from how you combine the frequency, intensity, and time of your exercise. A bigger dose gives you different benefits from a smaller dose.

Three days a week is the starting minimum in terms of frequency, going up to five. As your endurance and strength increase, you can do it more often. If you exercise vigorously, three days is enough. If your aerobic exercise is a comfortably-paced walk, you could build up to five or even seven days a week. Stick with moderate intensity—that is, where you can carry on a conversation while you exercise, a perceived-exertion level of no more than 6, or an exercise heart rate of no more than 75% of your age-predicted maximum heart rate. And the time you spend should be a minimum of thirty minutes accumulated low to moderate physical activity. To benefit your health, you can do the activity in three ten-minute bouts during the day. To improve cardiovascular fitness, you might have to carry on a bit longer each time.

When you start your exercise programme, it might help to take account of the accepted guideline that adults should accumulate thirty minutes of moderate physical activity on most days of the week. This is a goal, not necessarily your starting point. If you can manage two minutes spell of exercise once a day, at the beginning of your programme, you are likely to be able to reach the goal of thirty minutes, in three ten-minute sessions a day. This is enough to improve your health and for you to feel a good deal better.

When to Warm Up and Cool Down

Warm-Up

If you are going to exercise at an intensity that causes you to breathe harder or your heart to beat faster, you need to warm up first. A warm-up means that you do at least five minutes of a low-intensity activity to allow your heart, lungs, and circulation to gradually increase their work. If you are going for a brisk walk, warm up with five minutes of slow walking first. If you are riding on an exercise bicycle, warm up with five minutes of no resistance and no more than 60 rpm—revolutions per minute. In an aerobic exercise class, you will warm up with a gentle routine before getting more vigorous. Warming up reduces the risk of injuries, soreness, and irregular heartbeats.

Cool Down

At the other end, a cool-down period is important if you have exercised at an intensity that required you to breathe harder and your heart to beat faster, or if you felt warmer or perspired. Repeating the five-minute warm-up activity or taking a slow walk helps your muscles gradually relax and your heart and breathing to slow down. Gentle stretching and flexibility exercises during the cool-down can be effective for increasing motion because your muscles and joints are warm and more easily stretched. Also, stretching gently now helps reduce the muscle soreness and stiffness that may follow vigorous exercise. Make this a habit.

Endurance Exercises

Many activities can be aerobic and these build endurance. As you can carry on longer with any particular exercise, so your use of oxygen improves and your fitness develops. This chapter gives you some detail about a few of the more common ones, including walking, swimming, using an exercise bicycle and low-impact aerobics.

Walking

Walking can condition your heart and lungs, strengthen bones and muscles, relieve tension, control weight, and generally make you feel good. Walking is easy, inexpensive, safe and accessible. You can walk by yourself or with company, and you can take your exercise with you wherever you go. Walking is safer and puts less stress on the body than jogging or running. It's an especially good choice if you are older, have been sedentary, or have joint problems.

Most people with a chronic illness can walk as a fitness exercise. If you walk to the shops, to visit friends, and do household chores, then you'll probably be able to walk for exercise. Using a walking stick or walking aid need not stop you from getting into a walking routine. If you are in a wheelchair, use crutches, or experience more than mild discomfort when you walk a short distance, perhaps consider some other type of aerobic exercise, or consult a doctor or physiotherapist for help.

Be cautious during the first two weeks of walking. If you haven't been doing much for a while, ten minutes of walking may be enough. Build up your time with intervals of strolling. Each week increase the brisk walking interval by no more than five minutes until you are up to twenty or thirty minutes. Follow the frequency, duration, and intensity guidelines, and read these tips on walking before you start.

Walking Tips

- **Choose your ground.** Walk on a flat, level surface. Walking on hills, uneven ground, soft earth, sand, or gravel is hard work and often leads to hip, knee, or foot pain. Fitness trails, shopping centres, school tracks, streets with pavements, and quiet neighbourhoods are good places to get started.
- **Always warm up and cool down with a stroll.** It's important to walk slowly for three to five minutes to prepare your circulation and muscles for a brisk walk, and to finish up with the same slow walk to let your body slow down gradually. Experienced walkers know they can avoid shin and foot discomfort when they begin and end with a stroll.
- **Set your own pace.** It takes practice to find the right walking speed. To find your speed, start walking slowly for a few minutes,

then increase your speed to a pace that is slightly faster than normal for you. After five minutes, monitor your exercise intensity by checking your pulse, or using the perceived-exertion or talk methods. If you are above the range or feel out of breath, slow down. If you are below the range, try walking a little faster. Walk another five minutes and check your intensity again. If you are still below your exercise range, keep walking at a comfortable speed and simply check your intensity in the middle and at the end of each walk.

- **Increase your arm work.** You can also raise your heart rate into the "ideal" or target exercise range by increasing arm work. Bend your elbows a bit and swing your arms more vigorously. Alternatively, carry a one- or two-pound weight (·75 kg) in each hand. You can purchase hand weights for walking, hold a tin of food in each hand, or put sand, dried beans, or pennies in two small plastic bottles or socks. The extra work you do with your arms increases your intensity of exercise without forcing you to walk faster than you find comfortable.

Shoes

It's not necessary to spend a lot of money on shoes. Wear shoes of the correct length and width with shock-absorbing soles and insoles. Make sure they're big enough in the toe area. The "rule of thumb" is a thumb-width between the end of your longest toe and the end of the shoe. You shouldn't feel pressure on the sides or tops of your toes. The heel counter should hold your heel firmly in the shoe when you walk.

Wear shoes with a continuous crepe or composite sole in good repair. Shoes with leather soles and a separate heel don't absorb shock as well as the newer athletic and casual shoes. Shoes with laces or Velcro let you adjust width as needed and give more support than slip-ons. If you have problems tying laces, you could try Velcro closures or elastic shoelaces.

Many people like shoes with removable insoles that can be exchanged for more shock-absorbing ones. Insoles are available in sporting goods stores and shoe stores. When you shop for insoles, take your walking shoes with you. Try on the shoe with the insole to make sure that there's still enough room inside for your foot to be comfortable. Insoles come in sizes and can be trimmed with scissors for a neat fit. If your toes take up extra room, try the three-quarter insoles that stop just short of your toes. If you have prescribed inserts in your shoes already, ask your doctor about insoles.

Possible Problems

If you have pain around your shins when you walk, you may not be spending enough time warming up. Try some ankle exercises before you start walking. Start your walk at a slow pace for at least five minutes. Keep your feet and toes relaxed

Another common problem is sore knees. Fast walking puts stress on knee joints. To slow your speed and keep your heart rate up, try doing more work with your arms as suggested above. Do the Knee Strengthener and Ready-Go (Chapter 7, Exercises 17 and 19) in your warm-up to reduce knee pain.

Cramps in the calf and heel pain can be helped by doing the Achilles Stretch (Chapter 7 Exercise 21) before and after walking. A slow walk to warm up is also helpful. If you have circulatory problems in your legs, and experience cramps or pain in your calves while walking, alternate intervals of brisk and slow walking at whatever pace you can tolerate. Slow down and give your circulation a chance to catch up before the pain is so intense you have to stop. As you will see, such exercises may even help you to gradually walk farther with less cramping or pain. If this doesn't help, check with your doctor or physiotherapist for suggestions.

Maintain good posture. Remember the heads-up position in chapter 7 and keep your shoulders relaxed to help reduce neck and upper back discomfort.

Swimming

Swimming is another good endurance exercise. The buoyancy of the water lets you move your joints through their full range of motion. You can strengthen your muscles and cardiovascular system with less stress than on land. For most people with chronic illness, swimming is excellent exercise. It uses the whole body. If you haven't been swimming for a while, consider a refresher course.

To make swimming an endurance exercise, you will eventually need to swim continuously for twenty minutes. Use the frequency, duration, and intensity guidelines set out at the beginning of this chapter to build up your endurance. Try different strokes, modifying them or changing strokes after each lap or two. This lets you exercise all joints and muscles without overtiring any one area.

Swimming Tips

- The breast stroke and crawl normally require a lot of neck motion and may be uncomfortable if you have neck pain. To solve this problem, use a mask and snorkel so that you can breathe without twisting your neck.
- Chlorine can be irritating to eyes. Consider a good pair of goggles. You can even have swimming goggles made in your lens prescription.
- A hot shower or soak in a warm bath after your workout helps reduce stiffness and muscle soreness. Remember not to work too hard or get too tired. If you're sore for more than two hours, go easier next time.
- Always swim where there are qualified lifeguards if possible, or with a friend. Never swim alone.

Aquacise

If you don't like swimming, or are uncomfortable learning swimming strokes, you can walk laps in the pool or join the millions who are "aquacising"—exercising in water.

Aquacise is comfortable, fun, and effective as a flexibility, strengthening, and aerobic activity. The buoyancy of the water takes the weight off your hips, knees, feet, and back, so you might find it more attractive than walking. Exercising in a pool allows you a degree of privacy in doing your own routine, since no one can see you much below shoulder level. And no, it doesn't matter what you look like in a swimming costume!

Getting Started

Joining a water exercise class with a good instructor is an excellent way of getting started. Taking account of your own particular long-term condition, use your various professional consultants to work out how exercise in water can help you.

Cycling

Exercise bicycles offer the fitness benefits of cycling without the outdoor hazards. They're preferable for people who don't have the flexibility, strength or balance to be comfortable pedalling and steering on the road. Indoor use of exercise bicycles may also be preferable to outdoor cycling for people who live in a cold or hilly area.

The exercise bicycle is a particularly good alternative exercise. It doesn't put excess strain on your hips, knees, and feet, you can easily adjust how hard you work, and weather doesn't matter. Use the bicycle on days when you don't want to walk or do more vigorous exercise, or can't exercise outside.

Make it Interesting

The most common complaint about riding an exercise bike is that it's boring. If you cycle while watching television, reading, or listening to music, you can become fit without becoming bored. Maybe you could map out tours of places you would like to visit and then chart your progress on the map as you roll off the miles. Or set your bicycle time for the half-hour of soap opera or news that you watch every day. Alternately you could put on a DVD. Book racks that clip on to the handlebars make reading easy. Just pedalling and noticing your breathing can also, if you are patient, enable you to achieve a mental calm like meditation—have a look at chapter 5 for more on this.

Exercise Bicycle Checklist

- The bicycle is steady when you get on and off. The resistance is easy to set and can be set to zero. The seat is comfortable.
- The seat can be adjusted for full knee extension when the pedal is at its lowest point.
- Large pedals and loose pedal straps allow feet to move slightly while pedalling.
- There is ample clearance from the frame for knees and ankles.
- The handlebars allow good posture and comfortable arm position.

Cycling Tips

- Cycling uses different muscles from walking. Until your leg muscles get used to pedalling, you may be able to cycle for only a few minutes. Start off with no resistance. Increase resistance slightly every two weeks. Increasing resistance has the same effect as cycling up hills. If you use too much resistance, your knees are likely to hurt, and you'll have to stop too soon before you get the benefit of endurance.
- Pedal at a comfortable speed. For most people, 50–60 rpm is a good place to start. Some bicycles tell you the rpm, or you can count the number of times your right foot reaches its lowest point in a minute. As you get used to cycling, you can increase your speed. However, faster is not necessarily better. Listening to music at the right tempo makes it easier to pedal at a consistent speed. Experience will tell you the best combination of speed and resistance.
- Set your goal for twenty to thirty minutes of pedalling at a comfortable speed. Build up your time by alternating intervals of brisk pedalling with less exertion. Use your heart rate, perceived exertion or the talk test to make sure you aren't working too hard. If you're alone, try singing songs as you pedal. If you get out of breath, slow down.
- Keep a record of the times and distances of your "bike trips." You'll be amazed at how much you can do.
- On bad days, don't do nothing—keep your exercise habit going by pedalling with no resistance, at fewer rpm, or for a shorter period of time.

Other Exercise Equipment

If you have trouble getting on or off an exercise bicycle, or don't have room for a bicycle where you live, you might try a restorator or arm crank. Ask your physiotherapist or doctor, or phone a medical supplier.

A restorator is a small piece of equipment with foot pedals which can be attached to the foot of a bed or placed on the floor in front of a chair. It allows you to exercise by pedalling. You can adjust the resistance, and the leg length and knee bend. Depending on your symptoms, you may find the restorator to be an enjoyable first step in getting an exercise programme started.

Arm cranks are bicycles for the arms. They are mounted on a table. You'll need to work closely with a physiotherapist to set up your programme using one of these, because using only your arms for endurance exercise requires to be monitored differently from when you are using bigger leg muscles.

There is a wide variety of exercise equipment in addition to what has been mentioned so far. These include treadmills, self-powered and motor-driven rowing machines, cross-country skiing machines, mini-trampolines, and stair-climbing machines. Most are available in both commercial and home models. If you're thinking about exercise equipment, have your needs and your objectives clearly in mind. For cardiovascular fitness and endurance, you want equipment that will help you exercise as much of your body at one time as possible. The motion should be rhythmical, repetitive, and continuous. The equipment should be comfortable, safe, and not stressful on joints. If you're interested in a new piece of equipment, if possible try it out for a week or two before buying it.

Exercise equipment that requires you to use weights usually does not improve cardiovascular fitness unless individualised "circuit training" can be designed. A weight-lifting programme alone builds strength, but it can put excessive stress on joints, muscles, tendons, and ligaments. You will probably find that the flexibility and strengthening exercises in this book will help you safely achieve significant increases in strength as well as flexibility. Be sure that you consult your doctor or physiotherapist if you prefer to add strengthening exercises involving weights or weight machines to your programme.

Low-Impact Aerobics

Most people find low-impact aerobic dance an enjoyable and safe form of exercise. "Low impact" means that one foot is always on the floor and there is no jumping. However, low impact does not necessarily mean low intensity, nor do the low-impact routines protect all joints. If you go to a low-impact aerobic class, you'll probably need to modify what you do to suit yourself.

Getting Started

Start off by introducing yourself to your instructor and telling them that you may modify some movements to meet your needs. Say that you may need to ask for advice. You'll probably find it easier to start off with a newly formed class than to join an ongoing class. If you don't know people, try to make friends. Be open about why you may sometimes do things a little differently. You'll be more comfortable and may find others who also have special needs. Going a few times will make the class familiar as you settle in.

Most instructors use music or count to a specific beat and do a set number of repetitions. You may find that the movement is too fast or that you don't want to do as many repetitions. Modify the routine by slowing down to half-time, or keep up with the beat until you start to tire and then slow down or stop. If the class is doing an exercise that involves arms and legs and you get tired, try resting your arms and do only the leg movements, or just walk in place until you are ready to go again. Most instructors will be able to instruct you in "chair aerobics" if you need some time off your feet.

Some low-impact routines use a lot of arm movements done at or above shoulder level to raise heart rates. If this doesn't suit your condition, modify the exercise by lowering your arms or taking a rest break.

Feeling as though you look different from the group in a room walled with mirrors takes courage, conviction, and a sense of humour. The most important thing you can do for yourself is to choose an instructor who encourages everyone to exercise at her or his own pace and a class where people are friendly and having fun. Observe classes, speak to instructors, and participate in at least one class session before handing over money!

Aerobic Studio Tips

- **Wear shoes.** Many studios have cushioned floors and soft carpet that might tempt you to go barefoot. Don't! Shoes help protect the small joints and muscles in your feet and ankles by providing a firm, flat surface on which to stand.
- **Protect your knees.** Stand with knees straight but relaxed. Many low-impact routines are done with bent, tensed knees and a lot of bobbing up and down. This can be painful and is unnecessarily stressful. Avoid this by remembering to keep your knees relaxed—aerobics instructors call this "soft" knees. Watch in the mirror to see that you keep the top of your head steady as you exercise. Don't bob up and down.
- **Don't overstretch.** The warm-up at the beginning and the cool-down at the end of the session will have stretching and strengthening

exercises. Remember to stretch only as far as you comfortably can. Hold the position and don't bounce. If the stretch hurts, don't do it. Ask your instructor for a less stressful substitute, or choose one of your own.

- **Change movements.** Do this often enough so that you don't get sore muscles or joints. It's normal to feel some new sensations in your muscles and around your joints when you start a new exercise programme. However, if you feel discomfort doing the same movement for some time, change movements or stop for a while and rest.

Other Kinds of Exercise

Many exercise facilities have a variety of exercise opportunities—equipment rooms with cardiovascular machines, pools, and aerobic studios. If you have trouble with an hour-long aerobic class, see if you can join the class for the warm-up and cool-down and use an exercise bicycle or treadmill for your aerobic time. This routine can give you the benefits of both an individualised programme and group exercise.

Self-Tests for Endurance, or Aerobic Fitness

Often you just know you have made progress because you can do more and feel better. Some people could find it helpful to demonstrate that their exercise programme is making a measurable difference. It can be helpful, and quite fun, to try one or both of these aerobic fitness tests before you start your exercise programme. Not everyone will be able to do both tests, so pick one that works best for you. Record your results. After four weeks of exercise, do the test again and check your improvement. Measure yourself again after four more weeks.

Distance Test

Find a place to walk, cycle, swim, or water-walk where you can measure distance. A running track works well. On a street you can measure distance with a car. An exercise bicycle with an odometer provides the equivalent measurement. If you plan on swimming or water walking, you can count lengths of the pool.

After a warm-up, note your starting point and cycle, or swim, or walk as briskly as you comfortably can for five minutes. Try to move at a steady pace for the full time. At the end of five minutes, mark your spot or note the distance or laps and immediately take your pulse and rate your perceived exertion from 0 to 10. Continue at a slow pace for three to five more minutes to cool down. Record the distance, your heart rate, and your perceived exertion.

Repeat the test after several weeks of exercise. There may be a change in as soon as four weeks. However, it often takes eight to twelve weeks to see improvement.

Goal: To cover more distance or to lower your heart rate or to lower your perceived exertion.

Time Test

Measure a given distance to walk, cycle, swim, or water-walk. Estimate how far you think you can go in one to five minutes. You can pick a number of blocks, actual distance, or lengths in a pool.

Spend three to minutes warming up. Start timing and start moving steadily, briskly, and comfortably. At the finish, record how long it took you to cover your course, your heart rate, and your perceived exertion.

Repeat after several weeks of exercise. You may see changes in as soon as four weeks. However, it often takes eight to twelve weeks for a noticeable improvement.

Goal: To complete the course in less time or at a lower heart rate or at a lower perceived exertion.

Conclusion

Exercising to improve endurance has a central role in keeping muscles and other systems 'conditioned'. When faced by the challenges of a chronic condition the conditioned body (yours!) is much better able to resist and overcome them.

• • •

Suggested Further Reading

Cooper, Kenneth H. *The Aerobics Programme for Total Well Being: Exercise, Diet, Emotional Balance*. London: Bantam, 1989.

Gibson, Terry-Ann Spitzer. *Water Aerobics for Fitness and Wellness*, 3rd Edition. Belmont: Wadsworth, 2002

Krasavec, Joseph, and Grimes, Diane C. *Hydrorobics: A Water Exercise Program for Individuals of All Ages and Fitness Levels*. Champaign, Ill.: Human Kinetics Publishers, 1987.

Stewart, Gordon W. *Active Living: The Miracle of Medicine for a Long and Healthy Life*. Champaign, Ill.: Human Kinetics Publishers, 1995.

Weddington, Michael. *Aerobic Sports Log: A Revolutionary Graphical Log Book for the Health-Conscious Individual*. Griffin Publishing,1997.

CHAPTER 9

Communicating

"You just don't understand!"

How often has this statement, spoken or unspoken, summed up a frustrating verbal exchange? We all want other people to understand what we are trying to say. Feeling we are not understood is frustrating. Prolonged frustration can lead to depression, anger, and a sense of helplessness. Learning to live with a chronic condition can be frustrating enough, without adding communication problems.

Poor communication is a very large factor in poor relationships, whether they're between spouses, partners, family members or friends, colleagues at work, or doctors and patients. Even in casual relationships, poor communication causes frustration. We have all probably been irritable in a shop because of poor communication with a shop assistant. When you have a chronic illness, good communication is very important indeed. Your health care team, in particular, must "understand" you. As a self-manager, it will benefit you enormously to learn the skills necessary to make your communications as effective as possible.

This chapter suggests, as part of becoming an active self-manager of your life, that you review the way you use words and body language. It discusses how to improve the ways you communicate. If you feel unhappy, misunderstood or frustrated in some situations, (most people do!) start observing what you and others say, and notice the responses and the outcomes of particular conversations. Expressing feelings positively, asking for help and information, saying "no", minimising conflict, good listening—these are all skills that can be learned and developed.

Communication is an active process between people, each of whom continually adjusts to what is said and how it's said. Feelings are always stirring under what may seem to be the simplest of exchanges. Successful communication takes account of what underlies spoken words. Sometimes we get so caught up in our own feelings, perhaps our discomfort in asking for help, that we forget to make allowances for the possible discomfort of others. The more responsibility you can take for clarifying your own feelings and expressing them clearly, while allowing other people the freedom to express themselves in return, the more the lines of communication can be kept open. It is easy to fall into the trap of thinking "they should know . . ." They can't know until the message has been sent and received!

Expressing Your Feelings

There are complicated feelings attached to living with chronic illness. Consider the issues around working out what the problem is, in the example below.

John and Steve have agreed to go together to a football match. When John comes to pick up Steve, Steve is not ready and is not sure he wants to go because he is troubled with pain in his knees. The following conversation takes place.

John: Why do you always spoil my plans? At least you could have phoned and I could have asked my son to go with me.

Steve: You just don't understand. If you had pain like I do, you wouldn't be so quick to criticise. You don't think of anyone but yourself.

John: Well, I can see that I should just go by myself.

Neither John nor Steve has stopped to think about what is really bothering them or how they feel about it. Rather, they both blame the other for an unfortunate situation and the exchange finishes abruptly with no understanding.

The following is the same conversation in which both people take into account the need for clarity for each of them.

John: We have made plans and then at the last minute you are not sure you can go. I feel frustrated and angry. I don't know what to do—go on without you, stay here and change our plans, or just not make future plans.

Steve: When this pain plays up at the last minute, I get confused as well. I keep hoping I can go and so I don't I ring you because I don't want to disappoint you and anyway I really want to go. I keep hoping that my knees will get better as the day wears on.

John: I understand.

Steve: Let's go to the match. You can let me off at the gate before parking so I won't have to walk as far. Then I can take the steps slowly and be in our seats when you arrive. I do want us to keep making plans. In the future, I will let you know sooner if I think my arthritis is causing trouble.

John: Sounds good to me. I really do like your company and also knowing how I can help. It is just that being taken by surprise makes me angry.

John and Steve talk about the specific situation and how they feel about it. Neither blames the other.

Unfortunately, we are often in situations where the one person uses blaming communications. Perhaps we are caught not listening to what underlies their words, and resort to blaming communications ourselves.

Even in this situation, thoughtful communication can help.

Jan: Why do you always spoil my plans? At least you could have phoned. I am really tired of trying to do anything with you.

Sandra: I understand. When this asthma plays up at the last minute, I get confused. I keep hoping I can go and so don't phone you because I don't want to disappoint you and I really want to go. I keep hoping that I will get better as the day wears on.

Jan: Well, I hope that in future you will phone. I don't like being taken by surprise.

Sandra: I understand. If it's all right with you, let's go shopping now. I can walk a little way and rest in the coffee shop with my book while you carry on shopping. I do want us to keep making plans. In future, I'll let you know sooner if I think my asthma is causing trouble.

Only Sandra is using thoughtful communication. Jan continues to blame. The outcome, however, is still positive with both people accomplishing what they want.

If you can remain thoughtful in your conversations with others, you'll find that those around you who use blameful communication strategies will probably change to become more thoughtful themselves- it's infectious.

The following are some suggestions for keeping the lines of communication open and creating supportive relationships.

- When you find yourself with something you want to say, start by taking a few moments to review exactly what is bothering you and how you are feeling about it.
- Be clear. Use the facts of the particular situation. Avoid words like "always" and "never". For example, Sandra says, "When this asthma plays up at the last minute, I am confused. I keep hoping I can go and so don't phone you because I don't want to disappoint you and I really want to go. I keep hoping that I will get better as the day wears on."
- Show respect and regard for the other person. Be tactful and courteous. Avoid sarcasm. Don't put people down.
- Don't use language suggesting that you blame them, such as when Jan says, "Why do you always spoil my plans?" The use of the word "you" sounds accusing as if Jan blames Sandra, even if underneath she is just disappointed herself.
- Be open and honest about your feelings. Sandra does this when she talks about wanting to go, not wanting to disappoint Jan, and hoping that her asthma will get better.
- Don't turn yourself into a victim by *not* expressing your needs and feelings and then expecting others to act the way you think they "should" act.
- Try not to preach—don't tell people what they should do. Try not to demand that they do what you want.
- Work at using humour, but at the same time know when to be serious.
- Listen. Wait till the other person has finished speaking and give yourself a moment to register what is happening underneath their

words. Accept the feelings of others and try to understand them. Sometimes you need to think about what has been said. Rather than answer immediately, give yourself time to absorb it, with a reply like "I understand" or "I don't fully understand. Could you explain again?"

- Ask for explanations to sort out whether you are assuming correctly what underlies someone else's statements. Jan does not do this. She assumes that Sandra was being rude by not phoning her. She doesn't ask why she hasn't rung earlier. Assumptions—what you think people are feeling or thinking—often close down further communication if they are wrong.
- If you have in your head "they should know…" then you are probably making assumptions and might help everyone by asking a bit more.

"I" Messages

Many people are uncomfortable expressing feelings. This discomfort can be acute, and especially so if it means we might seem critical of the person we're talking to, or if we feel they might think less of us.

If emotions are high, attempts to express frustration can be laden with "you" messages that suggest blame. The other person feels under attack. They need to defend themselves and protective barriers go up. The person trying to express feelings, in turn, feels greater anxiety when faced with these defensive barriers and the situation escalates to anger, frustration, and bad feelings.

The use of "I", however, doesn't strike out or blame. It expresses how you feel, rather than suggesting that the other person is at fault for "making" you feel like that.

"You" message: Why are you always late? We never get anywhere on time.
"I" message: I get really upset when I'm late. It's important to me to be on time.

"You" message: There's no way you can understand how bad I feel.
"I" message: I'm not feeling well. I could really do with a little help today.

Watch out for hidden "you" messages. These are "you" messages with "I feel . . ." stuck in front of them.

"You" message: You always walk too fast.

Hidden "you" message: I feel angry when you walk so fast.

"I" message: I have a hard time walking fast.

The trick is to avoid the use of the word "you", and, instead, report your personal feelings using the word "I." Like any new skill, "I" messages take practice. Start by really listening, both to yourself and to others. Take some of the "you" messages you hear and turn them into "I" messages in your head. By playing this word game in your head, you'll be surprised at how quickly they become a habit in your own expressions.

There are some cautions to note when using "I" messages. First, they don't always work! at least, not immediately. Sometimes the listener has to have time to hear them. This is especially true if "you" messages and blaming have been the more usual ways of communicating. But keep trying. They really do work in the end.

Some people use "I" messages as a means of manipulation. If used in this way, problems can escalate. To be used effectively, "I" messages must report honest feelings.

Exercise—"I" Messages

Change the following statements into "I" messages. (Watch out for hidden "you" messages!)

You expect me to wait on you hand and foot!

Doctor, you never have enough time for me. You're always in a hurry.

You hardly ever touch me anymore. You haven't paid any attention to me since my heart attack.

You didn't tell me the side effects of all these drugs you're giving me or why I have to take them, doctor.

When using "I" statements seems difficult, try using this format: "When (here put in a specific situation) I (state your feelings)." For example, "When you don't ring, I worry."

"I" messages are an excellent way to express positive feelings and compliments! "I really appreciate the extra time you gave me today, doctor."

Minimising Conflict

Learning how to express our feelings through the use of "I" messages instead of "you" messages goes a long way to help reduce conflict in our relationships. We can also begin to manage conversations as they go along, to make sure they aren't knocked off course by the feelings that come up.

When a discussion gets off the topic and emotions run high, shift the focus back to what you agreed to talk about in the first place, and away from what is starting to happen between you. You might say something like, "We're both getting upset now and drifting away from the topic we agreed to discuss." Or, "I feel like we are bringing up other things than what we agreed to talk about, and I'm getting upset. Can we discuss these other things later and just talk about what we originally agreed on?"

Another tactic that prevents conflict or upset is to ask for time to think about things and respond later, when your emotions are not so intense. You might say, "I think I understand your concerns, but I need more time to think about it before I can respond." Or, "I hear what you are saying, but I am too frustrated to respond now. I need to find out more information about this before I can answer you."

Summarise what you think you have heard and ask for clarification to make sure you understand the other point of view. The scope for conflict is less if you have each made an attempt to stand back in see both sides. When you are thinking about a problem, you may also try switching roles. Try arguing the other person's position as thoroughly and thoughtfully as possible, to understand all the sides of an issue, as well as to respect and value the other's point of view. It helps develop tolerance and empathy for others as well.

You may not always find the perfect solution reach total agreement, but you can work toward an acceptable compromise. Find something that you can both agree to try for awhile. You can do it your way this time, and the other person's way the next time. Agree to part of what you want, and part of what the other person wants. Or, decide what you'll do, and what the other person will do in return. These are all forms of compromise that can help you through difficult times.

Asking For Help

Asking for help is hard. Many people feel awkward about asking for help or refusing help. The less independent you feel, the harder it can be to seem to admit dependence by showing you need help. Maybe it's difficult to admit to ourselves that we can't do things as easily as we could, another area where sorting out our own feelings first can take the pressure off a difficult conversation.

Try to avoid "hedging" your request: "I'm sorry to have to ask this . . ." "I know this is asking a lot . . ." "I hate to ask this, but . . . " Hedging may be meant to soften a request, but it tends to put the other person on the defensive: "Gosh, what's he going to ask for that's such a huge favour?"

Be specific about what help you are requesting. A general request can lead to misunderstanding, and the person can react negatively to insufficient information, which then leads to a further breakdown in communication. A specific request is more likely to lead to the desired goal or a positive result.

General request: I know this is the last thing you want to do, but I need help to move. Will you help me?

Reaction: Uh . . . well . . . I don't know. Um . . . can I get back to you after I check my other commitments? (probably next year!)

Specific request: I'm moving next week, and I'd like to move my books and the contents of the kitchen beforehand. Would you mind helping me load and unload the boxes in my car on Saturday morning? I think it can be done in one trip.

Reaction: I'm busy on Saturday morning, but I could give you a hand on Friday night, if you'd like.

Sometimes, you have to deal with refusing offers from people who genuinely want to be helpful. A well-worded "I" message can refuse the help tactfully, without embarrassing the other person. "Thank you for being so thoughtful, but today I think I can handle it myself. I'd like to be able to take you up on your offer another time, though."

Saying No

Perhaps you are the one being asked for help. Take time to gather full information before responding. Often our first feelings are negative if we don't know enough. "Help me move" can mean anything from carrying a wardrobe upstairs to lifting the phone to order a pizza. Sorting out specifics will aid the communication process. It is important to understand what the specific request is before responding. Asking for more information or paraphrasing the request will often help clarify it. Use a phrase such as "Before I answer . . . " to show you are finding out more before committing yourself.

Once you have decided to decline, acknowledge the importance of the request to the other person. They will see that you are rejecting the request, not them. Your turn-down shouldn't be a put-down. "You know, that's a worthwhile project you're doing, but I think it's beyond my capabilities this week." Again, specifics are the key. Be clear about the conditions of your refusal—is it for always, or just today or this week or right at this moment?

Accepting Help

Often our family or friends say "How can I help?" Our response is often "I don't know" while we are thinking "they should know. . . ." ! Be prepared to accept help with a specific answer. "It would be nice if we could go to the cinema once a month" or "Could you please take out the rubbish bag? I can't lift it." Most people can't read your mind, so you'll need to tell them what help you want and then thank them for it.

Listening

Most of us are much better talkers than listeners. Instead of listening to what the other person is saying and feeling we are often preparing a response—so we don't hear properly. There are some skills to work on.

- Listen to the words and tone of voice, and observe body language. Sometimes it's difficult to begin a conversation if there's a problem. There may be times when the words being used don't tell you there is something bothering this person. Is the voice wavering? Does he or she appear to be struggling to find "the right words"? Do you notice body tension? Does he or she seem distracted? If you pick up on some of these signs, this person probably has more on their mind than words are expressing.

- Let the person know you heard them. This may be a simple "uh huh." On many occasions the only thing the other person wants is acknowledgment, or just someone to listen, because sometimes merely talking to a sympathetic listener is helpful.
- Acknowledge the content and the underlying feeling of the remark. You can do this by restating the content of what you heard. "You are planning a trip." Or you can respond by acknowledging the emotions: "That must be difficult," or "How sad you must feel." When you respond on an emotional level, the results are often startling. You allow more expression of feelings and thoughts. Responding to either the content or emotion can help communication along by discouraging the other person from simply repeating what has been said.
- Respond by seeking more information. This is especially important if you are not completely clear about what is being said or what is wanted.

Body Language and Conversational Styles

Part of listening to what others are saying is observing how they say it. Even when we say nothing, our bodies are talking—even shouting! Research shows that more than half of what we communicate is conveyed through our body language rather than our words. Becoming aware of body language, facial expressions and tone of voice can help us deliver our own messages more clearly and understand better what other people say to us. What we do, how we look and how we sound should match the words we say, otherwise we send mixed messages and create misunderstandings. Look at the other person, whether you are speaking or listening. Remember to breathe. Check your body position—leaning forward slightly shows your interest, lounging back in a chair, closing your eyes, yawning, hiding behind a newspaper and leaving the room suggest inattention! Keep your facial expression relaxed and attentive. If you have something important to say, keep your body, your face and your voice firm, friendly and steady to support the assertive meaning of your words.

When you notice that the body language and words of others don't seem to match, ask for clarification to avoid misunderstandings. "I hear you saying that you would like to go with me to the family picnic, but you look tired and you're yawning as you speak. Would you rather stay home and rest, while I go alone?"

We all express ourselves differently. Our conversational style varies according to where we were born, how we were brought up, our occupation, our cultural background and our gender, and also to the immediate context of the exchange—a noisy place will affect how we converse, so will feeling under the weather. By acknowledging and accepting differences, we can open up honest communication and work co-operatively.

Getting More Information

Getting more information from another person is a bit of an art and there are several ways of doing it.

Ask for more. This is the simplest way to get more information. "Tell me more" will probably get you more, as will "I don't understand . . . please explain", "I would like to know more about . . ." ,"Could you put that another way?", "How do you mean?", "I'm not sure I got that", "Could you expand on that?"

Paraphrase. This is a good tool if you want to make sure you understand what the other person meant, not just what they said, but meant. Paraphrasing can either help or hinder effective communication, depending on the way it's worded. Use a question, not a statement—nobody likes to be told what they mean!

"Well, I don't know. I'm really not feeling up to par. This party will be crowded, there'll probably be smokers there, and I really don't know the hosts very well, anyway."

Paraphrased as a statement, it might look like this:

"So you're telling me you don't want to go to the party."

Paraphrased as a question:

"Are you saying that you'd rather stay at home than go to the party?"

The response to the first paraphrase might be anger—or even silence:

"No, I didn't say that! If you're going to be that way, I'll definitely stay at home."

"He just doesn't understand."

On the other hand, the response to the second paraphrase might be:

"That's not what I meant. I'm just feeling a little nervous about meeting new people. I'd appreciate it if you'd stay near me during the party. I'd feel better about it, and I might have a good time."

This promotes further communication, and the real reason for the doubt has been clarified. More information has emerged from the second paraphrase and no new information from the first one.

Be specific. If you want specific information, ask specific questions. We often speak in generalities.

Doctor: How have you been feeling?
Patient: Not so good.

The doctor doesn't have much in the way of information about the patient's condition. "Not good" isn't useful. Here's how the doctor gets more information:

Doctor: Are you still having those sharp pains in your left arm?
Patient: Yes. A lot.
Doctor: How often?
Patient: A couple of times a day.
Doctor: How long do they last?
Patient: A long time.
Doctor: About how many minutes, would you say?

Asking for specifics often produces information: "Can you be more specific about . . .?" "Are you thinking of something particular?" If you want to know "why", be specific about what it is. If you ask a specific question, you will be more likely to get a specific answer.

"Why?" is a general question and can set up a longer answer than you need. It may also suggest you are thinking of cause and effect, and the answer may be at a different level from the one you had in mind. Rather than "why", begin your responses with "who", "which", "when", or "where". These words prompt a specific response.

Sometimes we don't get the correct information because we don't know what question to ask. You may be seeking legal services from a Citizens' Advice Bureau. You phone and ask if they have a lawyer and hang up when the answer is no. If, instead, you had asked where you might get low-cost legal advice, you may have been given two or three contacts. Careful phrasing of questions is worth a bit of thought.

Communicating with Your Doctor

Making the health care system work better involves developing good communication with members of our health care team. This can be a challenge because many people feel intimidated or afraid to talk freely with their providers. Some professionals use unfamiliar medical words. Patients hesitate to ask what these words mean. Many people are afraid to share personal things about themselves because they don't really know and trust their providers. These fears block communication. Doctors may share the responsibility for poor communication because they often feel too busy or important to take the time to talk to and know their patients. They may be in a hurry and unaware of how their language or manner affects them.

While we do not have to become best friends with our providers, we should expect that they are attentive, caring, and able to explain things clearly to us. As a person with a chronic health problem, the relationship you have with your main healthcare provider must be looked on as a long-term one requiring regular work, much like a business partnership or even a marriage.

Your doctor will probably know more intimate details about you than anyone except perhaps your spouse or partner or parents. You, in turn, should be able to feel comfortable expressing your fears, asking questions that you may think are "stupid," and negotiating a treatment plan to satisfy you both, without feeling "put down" or that your doctor is not interested.

There are two things that will help to open, and keep open, the lines of communication with your doctor.

First, take account of how the doctor may feel. Too often, we expect them to act as a computer—a gigantic brain, stuffed with knowledge about the human body, especially ours, able to analyse, diagnose, make a prognosis, decide on treatment—and at the same time as a warm, caring person who makes you feel as though you're the only patient on their books

Actually, most doctors wish they were like that, too, but no doctor can be all things to all patients. They are human. They get headaches, they get tired, and they get sore feet. They have families who demand their time and attention, and they have to operate inside bureaucracies as formidable as the rest of us face.

Most doctors and other health care professionals entered the gruelling medical training system because they wanted to make sick people well. It is frustrating for them not to be able to cure someone with a chronic condition. They must take their satisfaction from improvements rather than cures, or even in maintenance of existing conditions rather than declines. Undoubtedly, you have been frustrated, angry, or depressed from time to time about your illness. Your doctor has probably felt the same about his or her inability to make you well. In this, you are truly partners.

Second, in this partnership between you and your doctor, there is limited time to build a relationship and establish good communication. You are likely to be short of time to discuss, to explain, to explore options. When time is short, anxiety can produce rushed exchanges, often leading to "you" messages, and messages that are just plain misunderstood—with no time to correct them.

A doctor is usually on a very tight timetable. This fact becomes painfully obvious to you when you have had to wait in the doctor's office because of an emergency that has delayed your appointment. Doctors try to stay on schedule, and sometimes patients and doctors alike feel rushed as a consequence. One way to help you to get the most from your visit with the doctor is to take P.A.R.T.

Prepare	**Ask**	**Repeat**	**Take action**

Prepare (and Prioritise)

Before visiting or ringing your doctor, prepare your "agenda". What are the reasons for your visit? What do you expect from your doctor?

Take some time to make a written list of your points. Be realistic. If you have thirteen different problems, it isn't likely that your doctor can adequately deal with that many concerns in one visit. Identify the main ones. Writing them down helps you remember them. Have you ever thought to yourself, after you walked out of the doctor's consulting room, "Why didn't I ask about . . . ?" or "I forgot to mention . . . ." Making a list beforehand helps you ensure your main concerns get addressed.

Mention your main concerns right at the beginning of the visit. Give your list to the doctor. If the list is long, expect that only two or three items will be addressed during this visit, and let your doctor know which items are the most important to you. Studies show that doctors allow an average of eighteen seconds for the patient to state his or her concerns before interrupting with focused questioning. Preparing your questions in advance will help you use your eighteen seconds well.

When the doctor asks, "What brings you in today?" you might say, "I have a lot of things I want to discuss on this visit". Looking at their watch, the doctor feels anxious. "But I know that we have a limited amount of time. The things that most concern me are my shoulder pain, my dizziness, and the side effects from one of the medicines I'm taking." The doctor is relieved because the concerns are focused and potentially manageable within the appointment time available.

Preparing for a visit involves more than just listing your concerns. You should be prepared to describe your symptoms concisely to the doctor (when they started, how long they last, where they are located, what makes them better or worse, whether you have had similar problems before, whether you have changed your diet, exercise, or medicines in a way that might contribute to the symptoms, and so on.). If a treatment has been tried, be prepared to report the effect of the treatment. If you have previous records or test results that might be relevant, bring them along. Tell your doctor about the trends (are you getting better or worse or are you the same?) and tempo (is it faster or slower?) of your problem, not just how you feel today. "In general I am slowly getting better, although today I do not feel well." In treating a chronic condition, the trends and tempo are very important.

Be as open as you can with your thoughts, feelings, and fears. Your doctor is not a mind reader. If you are worried, explain why: "I am worried that what I have may be contagious," or "My father had similar symptoms before he died," and so on. The more open you are, the more likely it is that your doctor can help you. If you have a problem, don't wait for the doctor to "discover" it. State it immediately. "I am worried about this mole on my chest."

Give your doctor feedback. If you don't like the way you've been treated by the doctor or someone else on the health care team, let your doctor know. If you were unable to follow the doctor's advice or had problems with a treatment, tell your doctor, so that adjustments can be made. Equally, most doctors appreciate compliments and positive feedback, but patients are often hesitant to praise their doctors. So, if you are pleased, let your doctor know.

Ask

Another key to effective doctor-patient communication is asking questions. Getting answers you understand and gathering information is one of the cornerstones of self-management. You need to be prepared to ask your doctor questions about diagnosis, tests, treatments, and follow-up.

- Diagnosis: Ask what's wrong, what caused it, if it is contagious, what is the future outlook (the prognosis), and what can be done to prevent it in the future.
- Tests: Ask if any medical tests are necessary, how they will affect your treatment, how accurate they are, and what is likely to happen if you are not tested. If you decide to have a test, find out how to prepare for the test and what it will be like. Also ask how you will get the results and when.
- Treatments: Ask about your treatment options including lifestyle change, medicines, surgery. Inquire about the risks and benefits of treatment and the consequences of not treating.
- Follow-up: Ask if and when you should phone in or return for a follow-up visit. What symptoms should you watch for, and what should you do if they occur?

You may wish to take some notes on important points during the visit or consider bringing along someone else to act as a second listener. Another set of eyes and ears may help you later recall some of the details of the visit or instruction. You may want to ask your doctor to have copies of any letters he or she writes about you; it is your right to have these letters.

Repeat

It is extremely helpful to repeat back briefly to the doctor some of the key points from the visit and discussion. These might include diagnosis, prognosis, next steps, treatment actions, and so on. This is to double-check that you clearly understood the most important information. Repeating back also gives the doctor a chance to correct any misunderstandings and miscommunications immediately. If you don't understand or remember something the doctor said, admit that you need to go over it again. You might say, "I'm pretty sure you told me some of this before, but I'm still confused about it." Don't be afraid to ask what you may consider a "stupid" question. These questions can often indicate something important.

Take Action

When the visit is ending, you need to understand clearly what to do next. When appropriate, ask your doctor to write down instructions or recommend reading material for more information on a particular subject.

If, for some reason, you can't or won't follow the doctor's advice, let the doctor know. "I didn't take the aspirin. It gives me stomach problems", or "I've tried to exercise before, but I can't seem to keep it up." If your doctor knows why you can't or won't follow advice, there may be an alternative. If you don't explain what stops you, it's difficult for your doctor to help

Before you leave the office, make sure you understand the next steps. For example, should you return for another visit? If so, why and when? If tests were taken, can you phone for the results? Are there any danger signs to watch for and report to your doctor?

Asking for a Second Opinion

Many people feel uncomfortable about asking their doctor for a second opinion about diagnosis or treatment. If you have had a long relationship with your doctor or you simply like them, you might sometimes worry that asking for another opinion could be interpreted by the doctor as questioning their competence. It is a rare doctor whose feelings will be hurt by a sincere request for another opinion. Even if your condition is not particularly complicated, asking for a second opinion is a perfectly acceptable, and often expected, request. Doctors prefer a straightforward request and asking in a non-threatening "I" message will make this task simple: "I'm still feeling confused and uncomfortable about this treatment. I feel another opinion might help me feel more reassured. Can you suggest someone I could consult?" In this way, you have expressed your own feelings without suggesting that the doctor is at fault. You have also confirmed your confidence in him or her by asking that he or she suggest the other doctor. You aren't bound by his or her suggestion. You may choose anyone you wish for a second opinion.

Give Positive Feedback to Your Providers

Your providers need to know how satisfied you are with your care. If you don't like the way you have been treated by any of the members of your health care team, let this person know. In the same way, if you are pleased with your care, let your providers know. Everyone appreciates compliments and positive words of feedback, especially members of your health care team. They are human, and your praise can help nourish and console these busy, hardworking professionals. Letting them know that you appreciate their efforts is one of the best ways to improve your relationship with them!

In summary, the box below gives examples of some words that can help or hinder.

Working with the Health and Social Care System

The National Health Service is going through many changes. This can lead to problems both for the patients as well as for the health and social care professionals.

Words That Help	Words That Hinder
at this moment	never
at this time	always
at this point	every time
today	constantly
I	you
who	obviously
which	why
where	but
when	
how do you mean	
please explain	
tell me more	
I don't understand	

Your doctor or other care professionals may be just as upset as you when the system does not work well. New ways are being developed to get patients more involved in improving the NHS. If you are unhappy with the system, you can now do a lot more. You can find out how local decisions are made and who makes them. Each Primary Care Trust (PCT) board has a patient representative. You can contact them by letter or phone. If you have problems with your local GP surgery, you can contact the Practice Manager.

In every NHS hospital you now have the PALS (Patient Advocacy and Liaison Service) staff with whom you can discuss your problems. Look out for opportunities in your area to contribute to this new agenda in active citizenship. The most important thing you can do is to work in partnership with your care professionals so that together you can find ways to make the system work well for you. You can also contact local Patients Forums or even become a member of a local Forum.

In many countries, health care has become more complex, and in many cases, it has become big business. There are many more types of health care providers working with many more patients. They play supporting roles in these organisations and share in the same frustrations. It has become impossible for one provider to know everything about their patients, and patients often see more than one provider. In addition, there are more tests to take and other health professionals with whom to consult, such as registered dietitians and physical therapists and, of course, there are many more drugs. Health care may be better and more thorough, but getting that care is much more complicated.

A website called NHS Choices (www.nhs.uk) may be helpful for you here. It is designed to give as much information as possible about different diseases and how and where to get the best treatments.

If you are unhappy with your health care system, don't just fume quietly—do something about it. Find out who is running the organisation and how decisions are made. Then share your feelings in a constructive way by letter, phone, or email. Most health care systems want to keep you as a patient, and therefore usually respond when patients push enough. The problem is that the people who make the decisions tend to isolate themselves from the patients, so it is easier to express our feelings to the receptionist, nurse, or doctor. Unfortunately, these people have little or no power in the system. They can, however, tell you who to ring or write to. The more closely you can form a partnership with your providers, the better able all of you together will be to make the system more responsive.

The following are a few examples of practical communication with the health care system.

- "I hate the phone system." Or, "I hate it when I call and all I get is an automated message." Often, when we call for an appointment or information, we are routed through an automated phone system. This is frustrating, and unfortunately there is not much we can do about it. However, phone systems tend not to change too often, so if you can note or memorise the numbers or keys to press, you can move more quickly through the system. Once you do get through, ask if there is a way to do this faster next time. Is there another number? Is there a "best" time of the day to call?

- "It takes too long to get an appointment." As our systems get busier, this is often a problem. Ask for the first available appointment. Take it. Then ask how you can learn about cancellations. In some systems they will be happy to call you to fill an appointment slot. In others, you may have to call them once or twice a week to check. Ask the person making the appointment what you should do. They might also give you a telephone number so that you can reach them directly. No matter how frustrated you are, though, be polite. You are more likely to get what you want!

- "I have so many doctors; I do not know who to ask for what." One of those doctors has to be in charge, so find out which one. Ask each doctor you see who is in charge of coordinating your care. When you get a name, it is most likely your primary care doctor or GP. Ring them to confirm that they are doing the coordination. Ask how you can help. Let the coordinating doctor know when someone else orders a test or new medication, especially if there is no electronic medical record.

- "So what is an electronic medical record?" More and more of your medical information is being put on a secure computer that can be accessed by any of your providers—as long as they are in the same system. You should know what information is on the system. Sometimes it is just test results; sometimes it is test results and medication information; sometimes it is everything that is known about you. An electronic medical record is just like a paper record—it does no good if your providers don't read it. When you have a test, the doctor ordering the test will be informed of the test result. Tell other doctors who see you to read the results. Learn about the medical records system that contains your information so you can help your providers use it more effectively.

You have a right to a copy of almost everything in your record. It's a good idea to ask for copies of all your test results so that you can carry them with you from one provider to the next. In this way, you also know that they will not get lost in the system.

- "I have to wait too long in the waiting room or the examination room." Emergencies happen sometimes, and this can cause a wait. More often, you are at the mercy of an inefficient system. Before leaving home, ring your doctor and ask how long you will have to wait. Explain that you will be there, but not until about fifteen minutes before the doctor expects to see you. You can also show up and ask about the wait. Go to the visit prepared to wait; bring a book or something else to do while you wait. Rather than getting upset, let the receptionist know that you are going to step out for a while and that you will return at a specified time.

- "I don't have enough time with the doctor." This is a system problem. The doctor is usually told how much time they can have with each patient. When making the appointment, ask for the amount of time you want, especially if this is more than ten or fifteen minutes—be prepared to make a case for more time. You can also ask for the last appointment in the day. You may have to wait a while, but at least the doctor will not be rushed by having to see another patient. If you request more time than is allotted, you make other people wait. It may not seem much at first glance but a doctor often sees thirty patients a day. If each one takes five extra minutes, this means that the doctor has to work an extra two and a half hours that day. That little bit of extra time really adds up.

- "I can't get my doctor on the phone. She won't call back." Ask your doctor how to best communicate directly with them. This might be by email, or they may give you their private number or a number of a nurse practitioner with whom they work. The more a doctor trusts you not to abuse the privilege of having personal contact information, the more likely you are to be able to establish direct communication.

If you are given this privilege, use it wisely. Usually patients don't call the doctor directly for a repeat prescription. Use the system for doing this. If you do need to contact the doctor about medication, send a message or a note with a return envelope via the nurse, two to three weeks before your prescription runs out.

> Contact your doctor directly only for the important things.
>
> By the way, a medical emergency is certainly important, but don't waste time trying to contact your doctor. Ring 999, or go to a hospital accident and emergency department.

If something in the health care system is not working for you, ask how you can help to make it work better. Very often, if you learn the workings of the system, you move towards solving your problems. No-one would disagree with you if you think that things should not be like this and that it is not fair to place such burden on the patient. Health systems should all change, as some are doing, to be more responsive and patient-friendly. In the meantime, systems are run by individuals. By learning the system and by communicating well with the individuals in it, you can manage your relationships to get the best care the system can provide.

• • •

Suggested Further Reading

Beach, Wayne A. *Conversation About Illness: Family Preoccupations with Bulimia*. Hove, Sussex: Lawrence Erlbaum, 1996.

Beck, Aaron. *Love Is Never Enough: How Couples Can Overcome Misunderstandings, Resolve Conflicts, and Solve Relationship Problems Through Cognitive Therapy*. London: Harper Collins, 1989.

Egan, Gerard. *The Skilled Helper*. 7th Edition. Belmont, Cal.: Wadsworth, 2001.

Gabor, Don. *Talking with Confidence*. London: Sheldon Press, 1999.

Hargie, Owen. *A Handbook of Communication Skills*. 2nd Edition. London: Routledge, 1996.

Jones, J. Alfred, Gary L. Kreps, and Gerald M. Phillips. *Communicating with Your Doctor: Getting the Most out of Health Care*. Cresskill, N.J.: Hampton Press, 1995.

McKay, Matthew, Martha Davis, and Patrick Fanning. *Messages: The Communication Skills Book*. Oakland, Calif.: New Harbinger Publications, 1983.

CHAPTER 10

Sex and Intimacy

Many couples who live with a chronic health condition, with either one partner or both having a condition, may face a challenge in keeping this important part of their relationship alive and well. Fear of hurting someone or causing a health emergency can dampen desire in one or both partners. Fear of making symptoms worse can be frustrating. Sex, after all, is supposed to be joyful and pleasurable, not frightening or uncomfortable!

Sex is more than the act of sexual intercourse; it is also the sharing of physical and emotional sensuality. There is a special intimacy when we make love. Believe it or not, having a chronic health problem can actually improve your sex life by making you experiment with new types of physical and emotional stimulation for you and your partner. Exploring sensuality with your partner can open communication and strengthen your relationship as well. Additionally, natural "feel-good" hormones, called "endorphins," are released in our bloodstreams when we have sex.

Obstacles

It is intercourse itself that can be an obstacle for many people with chronic conditions, because of the physical demands it places on our bodies. Increased heart rate and faster breathing can tax someone with limited energy or breathing or circulatory problems. Some people are unable to find a sexual position that is completely comfortable, or they find pain, shortness of breath, or fatigue during sex to be so distracting that it interferes with their enjoyment of sex or their ability to have an orgasm. If you can't, and they can, you may feel resentful and they may feel guilty. If you avoid sex because of this without clarifying the situation, your relationship is likely to suffer. Everything suffers because communication stops.

People are afraid, too, that someone who has had a heart attack or a stroke might have another episode during sex. People with breathing difficulties worry that sex is too strenuous and will bring on an attack of coughing and wheezing. Their partners may also be anxious about this, fearing as well that they could be responsible for causing extra suffering and even death. Some people believe they are physically unattractive as a result of their disease. If self-image and self-esteem are low, for anyone, it can be a subtle barrier to sexual relationships and to sexual satisfaction. Someone who is partly paralysed, or who has put on weight as a side-effect of their medicine, may feel limited by their symptoms. Functional problems like incontinence or the appearance of swollen joints may erode the person's sense of being a whole, functioning being.

Anyone with a chronic condition will have experienced fear that it will get worse, or even life-threatening. Health problems do get in the way of the activities that we want and need to do. When sex is the activity, we have a difficult problem. Not only are we anxious about an important, pleasurable part of our own life, but we probably feel guilty and anxious about our partner as well. Our partner may even feel more fearful and guilty than we do—afraid that he or she might hurt us during sex, but at the same time, guilty for maybe feeling resentful. This dynamic can cause serious problems in a relationship, and the stress and depression these problems cause can even cause more symptoms.

People with these or other obstacles to a happy sex-life may avoid sexual situations, and "try not to think about it." Denying the presence of sexual energy is the same as, for example, denying the energy of anger—it often leads to depression, and depression leads to lack of interest in sex, and that leads to depression . . . a vicious circle. Sorting out the roots of any symptoms, emotional or physical, is part of what this book aims to help you with—actively tackling this aspect of your life is as possible as taking control in any other. You can feel better. For more on depression and how to help yourself overcome it, see chapter 4.

Sensuality

It's helpful to spend more time on sensuality or foreplay and less on actual intercourse. By concentrating on ways to arouse your partner and give pleasure while in a comfortable position, your intimate time together can last longer and be very satisfying. Many people enjoy climax without intercourse; others may wish to climax with intercourse. For some, climax may not be as important as sharing pleasure and they are satisfied without an orgasm. No matter how or if climax is reached, uncomfortable symptoms can be minimised if we concentrate on foreplay and sensuality rather than intercourse itself. There are many ways to enhance sensuality during sexual activity. In sex, as in other things, our minds and bodies are linked and we can increase the sexual pleasure we experience in both.

The largest sensual organ of our bodies is the skin. It is rich with sensory nerves. The right touch on almost any area of our skin can be very erotic. Fortunately, sexual stimulation through touch can be done in just about any position. It can be further enhanced with the use of oils, flavoured lotions, feathers, fur gloves—turn your imagination loose on this one! Just about any part of the skin can be an erogenous zone, but the most popular are the mouth, ear lobes, neck, breasts—for both sexes, navel area, hands—fingertips if you are giving pleasure, palms if you are receiving pleasure, wrists, small of the back, buttocks, toes, and insides of the thighs and arms. Experiment with the type of touch—some find a light touch arousing, others prefer a firm touch. It is not necessary to limit yourself to your hands, either. Many people become very aroused when touched with the lips, tongue, or sex toys.

Overcoming Fear During Sex

There is an estate agents' maxim: "The three things to consider when buying a house are location, location, location". Well, for sex, they are communication, communication, communication! The best way to address the fears of both partners is to confront them and address them through talking and listening. Learning new positions and ways to increase sensuality will help, but they are not going to be enough without good communication. People with (or without) long-term conditions need to be able to give and receive honest and open information, and to reassure themselves and each other that each has the other's best interests at heart. Agreeing to share the process of opening up communication is the first step in dealing with fear, anxiety and the practical problems.

Have a look at chapter 9, where you and your partner may find some help with communication skills. If these techniques are new, give them time. Any new skill takes patience and practice. One possibly difficult conversation isn't enough—agreeing to raise the subject again, and talking some more, will make subsequent attempts easier and more productive. As you and your partner get comfortable talking about sex, you can go about finding solutions to the problems you perceive.

Look also at the problem-solving techniques in chapter 2. It may seem a bit odd to think of the private intimacies of a sexual relationship in terms of goal-setting and problem-solving! However, while you may not sit down and write it all out, it can really help you as an individual and both of you as a couple to identify what you want, what's getting in the way, and what to do about it.

A sense of humour helps, too.

Overcoming Symptoms During Sex

A first self-management step is to identify which symptom causes you what problem, and to develop an action plan around the available options.

One option might be to time taking your medicine to be at peak effectiveness when you want to have sex. Of course, this involves planning ahead!

Another option is consider a change of medication. If you take a narcotic-type painkiller, for example, or one containing muscle relaxants or tranquillisers, you may find that your sensory nerves are dulled along with your pain. Obviously, it would be counter-productive to dull the nerves that will give you pleasure. Thinking may also be muddled due to the medication and make it more difficult to focus. Some medications can also make it difficult for a man to achieve an erection.

A further option at this point would be to approach one of your consultants, your doctor or pharmacist, for information about possible timing or alternatives if this is a problem for you. Different long-term conditions cause different sorts of problems. These problems are worth mentioning to your doctor. It's unlikely that your problem is unique. Your doctor has probably heard about it before and may have some solutions to suggest.

To keep both partners comfortable it is important to experiment with physical positions for sex. Everybody is different and no one position is good for everyone. Try things out—before you and your partner are too aroused to change course. Placing pillows strategically, or sitting on a chair, whatever you both agree. Anyway, it may be a good idea to change positions periodically during sex if one position causes difficulty after a while. This can be fun, not a nuisance. Stopping to rest is fine!

An option involving using your mind to manage your symptoms—have another look at chapter 5—is to become the world's best fantasist. What goes on in our minds can be extremely arousing. If it weren't, there would be no strip clubs, pornography, or even romantic novels. Most people engage in sexual fantasy at some time or another. There are probably as many sexual fantasies as there are people, and any are fine to indulge in mentally. If you discover a fantasy you and your partner share, you can play it out in bed, even if it is as simple as a particular saying you or your partner like to hear during sex. Engaging your mind during sexual activity can be every bit as arousing as the physical stimulation. It is also useful when symptoms during sex interfere with your enjoyment.

To be really good at something, you have to train for it, and this is no exception. If you develop some sexual fantasy that you can indulge in when needed, making it vivid in your mind, you can call it up and concentrate on it. Picturing yourself and your partner making love while you actually are can keep your mind in the pleasure of the present. You won't be thinking about your symptoms. You will need to practise this! Using the power of your mind in this area may not have been your habit in the past. You can start with any guided imagery tape or script—not necessarily about sex—such as the one in chapter 5, working to make it more vivid each time you practise. Gradually make your focus an erotic one. Start with just picturing the images. When you get good at that, add and dwell on colours. Then, in your mind, look down to your feet as you walk. Listen to the sounds around you. Concentrate on the smells and tastes in the image and feel your skin being touched by a breeze or mist. Finally, feel yourself touch things in the image. Work on one of the senses at a time. Become good at one before going on to another. You can invent your own sexual fantasy and gradually make it real—picture it, hear it, smell it, and feel it. You can begin your fantasy by picturing yourself setting your symptoms aside. The possibilities are limited only by your imagination! Learning to call on this level of concentration can help you focus on the moment. Really focusing on your physical and emotional sensations during sex can be powerfully erotic. If your mind wanders, which is quite normal, gently bring it back to the here and now.

There are not many BUTs—but it is important not to try to overcome chest pain in this way. Chest pain should not be ignored. Get help straight away if you suffer from an episode of chest pain.

Total abstention from sex is an option. In other words, you might decide you will abstain from sex altogether because symptoms get so much in the way of your enjoyment. An advantage of proper action-planning is that you avoid drifting into major decisions without proper information-gathering and consideration. Since such a decision necessarily involves both partners, talking to each other, to be sure that both of you understand how things are, is a good idea at this stage.

It may be helpful to get outside help with such a conversation from a trained consultant. Someone who knows how to facilitate good communication can be a useful third person. It could be an unusual and difficult step for one or both partners to speak to each other in front of someone else about anything so private, but an agreement to keep talking can really be helped by a neutral professional. Both partners are likely to be exploring their own complicated and deep feelings as well as communicating them to each other, and a trained listener can help sort out how to handle one thing at a time.

Sex as Exercise

Physical activity is a big step towards living a healthy life with a chronic condition. Sex is physical activity and although not much discussed in gym programmes, undoubtedly contributes to your quota of exercise! From a practical point of view—as for any vigorous activity it's a good idea to do some warm-up exercises. (Yes, seriously!) Look at some of the stretching exercises from chapter 7. Sex can be good exercise, and increasing your fitness around walking, swimming, cycling, and so on, can have a very good effect on your sex life. Suppleness, stamina, increased aerobic fitness and extra breath are all very useful for good sex. Also, don't over-do it! Learn your limits and pace yourself, just as you would with any other physical activity.

A problem around intimacy—complex, private and profound as it may be—is just another problem associated with your chronic condition, like fatigue, pain and other physical limitations. Once you have identified the problem, it can be approached in the same way as you have approached your other problems as a self-manager. Chronic health problems need not mean the end of sex. Like other areas of change in your life, it may take courage and energy to tackle difficulties, but by talking with your partner, being willing to try out new ideas and maintaining your sense of humour, difficult relationships can be improved and even good sex can get better.

• • •

Suggested Further Reading

Association to Aid the Sexual and Personal Relationships of People with a Disability (SPOD), 286 Camden Road, London, N7 0BJ Tel 020 7607 8851. Contact for list of publications.

Ornstein, Robert, and David Sobel. *Healthy Pleasures*. Reading, Mass.: Addison-Wesley, Longman Inc., 1990.

Silverburg, Cory, Kaufman, Miriam, Odette, Fran. *The Ultimate Guide to Sex & Disability: For All of Us Who Live with Disabilities, Chronic Pain and Illness*. San Francisco: Cleis Press, 2004.

CHAPTER 11

Making Your Wishes Known: Advance Directives for Health Care

Thinking about the future is part of being a good self-manager. Deciding what we want to do if we lose the mental capacity to control our lives, before it actually happens, takes courage and determination. Deciding on our wishes around our death, before we absolutely have to, is equally challenging.

As a self-manager, tackling these decisions is part of actively taking control of your life. The process of working out what you want and don't want, as the first stage in action-planning, involves facing feelings most of us tend to avoid tackling. Practical matters require you to talk to those around you, including, perhaps, those you would like to spare possible pain. But once you have confronted the issues, discussed, decided, recorded and communicated your wishes, you will be rewarded by increased peace of mind.

This chapter looks at some documents to help in those situations which most of us will face. Some of them may have confusing or similar titles, so each document is explained.

Ordinary Power of Attorney

An ordinary Power of Attorney allows you to appoint another person to act for you in relation to your property and affairs when you are still capable of acting for yourself, but choose not to. You can choose to make a general power, which will cover most decisions or a specific power to do specific things; for example, if you go on holiday while you are selling your house then you may give your solicitor Power of Attorney to complete the sale on your behalf. The ordinary power cannot be used if you lack mental capacity.

Enduring Power of Attorney

An Enduring Power of Attorney is different as it continues to apply when you are not mentally capable of acting on your own. It was possible to make Enduring Power of Attorney documents (EPAs) until October 2007. An Enduring Power of Attorney is a document that appoints another person to act on your behalf in handling your property and financial affairs when you are able but also if you are mentally incapable of doing so yourself.

In other words, it allows someone else to make decisions for you, pay bills, even sell your home if you are unable to make decisions yourself (e.g. when in a coma or mentally not competent).

Since October 2007 it has not been possible to make an Enduring Power of Attorney as the Lasting Power of Attorney has replaced it. People with an existing EPA may choose to cancel the power and instead make a Lasting Power of Attorney, if there is need to change it; for example you have changed your mind about the person you have appointed. It is important to remember that Enduring Power of Attorney documents made before October 2007 are still valid, and your wishes will still be respected.

Lasting Power of Attorney

Lasting Power of Attorney (LPA) was brought in under the Mental Capacity Act 2005. The major difference between Lasting Power of Attorney (LPA) and the previous Enduring Power of Attorney is that there are two types of LPAs. A welfare power, where you can choose someone to make health and welfare decisions on your behalf, and a property and affairs power where the attorney can make decisions relating to your property and affairs. The welfare power can only be used when you lack capacity to make welfare, including medical decisions. The property and affairs power can be used when you have mental capacity (unless you restrict this in the power) as well as when you lack mental capacity to make such decisions.

The Mental Capacity Act starts from the belief that every adult has the right to take decisions, where they have mental capacity to do so, unless proven otherwise. Adults have the right to be supported in the decisions they make when they are able, even if the decisions seem unwise. Diagnosis of a particular medical condition e.g. dementia does not affect these rights, which means that the individual can make a decision that they are mentally able to make.

You may if you wish choose to name different attorneys for different LPAs. An attorney will only be able to make decisions for you regarding life-saving treatments if you write this into the document. An attorney will not be able to make decisions that are not in your best interest.

When choosing an attorney, there are a number of things to consider. It is possible to choose a relative, friend or an independent person, but they need to be ready and prepared emotionally when the time comes to carry out your wishes. As Lasting Power of Attorney gives someone else you nominate so much power it is very important you as the 'donor' trust the person. You may choose one attorney or more than one. If you have more than one attorney you must choose whether they act jointly (that is they must act together and cannot make decisions independently of the other) or jointly and severally (that is they act together but can also act separately if they so wish). There is no right or wrong answer, although joint attorneys acting jointly will afford you the best protection for the future against abuse, although if one of the attorneys were unable to act or were removed, the remaining attorney could no longer act, unless you made provision for a replacement.

It is best to set up a Lasting Power of Attorney with the help of a solicitor or Law Centre. Lasting Power of Attorney documents must be set up using an official form, and you must be able to make decisions when you set one up. An independent person must also certify in the form that you understand what you are doing. These documents must be registered with the Office of the Public Guardian who can provide further advice (contact details are at the end of this chapter).

Independent Mental Capacity Advocate (IMCA) Service

This Service, introduced under the Mental Capacity Act 2005, will support and represent people who do not have the capacity to make decisions where there is no one such as a relative, carer or friend to consult. It is for cases where a person lacks capacity to make decisions about serious medical treatment or long-term hospital or care home accommodation moves. IMCAs cannot be instructed if a person has an existing Enduring Power of Attorney or Lasting Power of Attorney.

Deciding What You Want: "Living Wills"

We all have feelings about our own death. Death may be feared, accepted, welcomed or, all too often, pushed aside to be thought about later. In the back of our minds, most of us have ideas about how and when we would like to die. For some of us, life is so important that we feel everything should be done to sustain it. For others, life is important only so long as we can be active participants. For many people, the issue isn't really death but, rather, dying. An eighty-year-old who dies skiing may be said to have had a "good" death, whereas her death in a nursing home unaware of her surroundings might be perceived as less "good" and not what we would wish for ourselves. The first step towards deciding what you want is to spend some time exploring your own innermost feelings.

While none of us can have absolute control over our own deaths, dying, like the rest of our lives, is something we can help manage. That is, we can have input, make decisions, and probably add a great deal to the quality of our death. Thoughtful self-management can lessen the negative impacts of our death on our survivors, too. This section of the chapter deals with information to help you manage better some of the legal issues around death. You can do this by drawing up what is commonly known as a "living will". This is different from a last will and testament, which applies after death. A living will applies when you are still alive.

It's important that your living will is entered into your medical notes so that in an emergency it is found and acted upon. Consider sending a copy to your doctor, a copy to any hospital which is treating you and a copy to your nearest relatives. If your living will is verbal, make sure close relatives or friends are aware.

A living will can be in the form of an Advance Statement stating your wishes, or an Advance Decision to refuse certain kinds of medical treatment.

Living Wills in the Form of Advance Statements

Advance Statements are general written statements about the kind of treatment you would or wouldn't like to receive should you lose mental capacity in the future. They are not legally binding on the health professional, but an opportunity for you to make a general statement of your values. The health care team will have to take your wishes into account when deciding on the right treatment for you.

Family and friends can indicate how your Advance Statement contains evidence of your wishes. You can make your views known verbally, for example, when discussing treatment with a health care professional; but having it written down makes things clearer for everyone.

Living Wills in the Form of Advance Decisions

A valid Advance Decision (sometimes referred to as an Advance Directive) will usually apply when you are close to death. The Decision indicates your wish to refuse all or some forms of medical treatment, in specified circumstances, at a time when you lack mental capacity to make that medical decision. You cannot use it to request treatment, or to ask for your life to be ended. Neither can you use it to nominate someone else to make decisions on your behalf.

Until 2007 Advance Directives, stating your wishes about the life-saving treatments you want or don't want to receive were valid under Common Law. From this date, living wills in the form of Advance Decisions are valid legal documents under the Mental Capacity Act 2005. They are viewed in law in the same way as a refusal of treatment by a person with capacity and the treatment cannot lawfully be given.

Advance Decisions are therefore binding on the health professional as long as they have been set up properly. An Advance Decision must:

- Be made by a person who is 18 or over and has the capacity to make it
- Specify the treatment to be refused (it can do this in lay terms)
- Specify the circumstances in which this refusal would apply
- Not have been made under the influence or harassment of anyone else
- Not have been modified verbally or in writing since it was made

Any refusal of life-saving treatment will need to be in writing. It will need to be signed and witnessed, and include an express statement that the decision stands "even if life is at risk".

Advance Decisions cannot be used to refuse basic nursing care (for example, washing), pain relief, food or drink or other appropriate care.

As with Advance Statements, it is a good idea to bear in mind that new drugs or treatments may be introduced in the future, so you may wish to allow for new treatments, even if refusing a current one.

It's important to note that diagnosis of a particular condition such as Alzheimer's or mental illness will not affect your right to make a living will. What matters is that you understand what you are doing when you make the living will, can retain that information and use it to guide your decision-making. You should also be able to understand the reasonable foreseeable consequences of what would happen if you did not make an advance decision or if you made it in different terms.

A doctor might not act on an Advance Decision if:

- The person has done anything clearly inconsistent with the advance decision which affects its validity (for example, a change in religious faith)
- The current circumstances would not have been anticipated by the person and would have affected their decision (for example, a recent development in treatment that radically changes the outlook for their particular condition)
- The document isn't clear about what should happen
- The person has been treated under the Mental Health Act and the advance decision relates to treatment for the mental disorder the person is suffering from.

A doctor can also apply treatment if there is doubt or a dispute about the validity of an Advance Decision, and the case has been referred to the court. This is why it is so important to set up a living will properly.

A living will becomes effective immediately after you have signed it, but it can be changed or cancelled at any time by you. It cannot be changed or contested by family, friends or any others including health professionals as long as it is valid and applies in the circumstances.

Expressing Your Wishes in Detail

For a living will one of the most important things is deciding what you want to put in it. For example:

I do not want my life to be prolonged and I do not want life-sustaining treatment to be provided or continued:
(1) if I am in an irreversible coma or persistent vegetative state; or
(2) if I am terminally ill and the application of life-sustaining procedures would serve only to artificially delay the moment of my death; or

(3) under any other circumstances where the burdens of the treatment outweigh the expected benefits. I want my agent to consider the relief of suffering and the quality as well as the extent of the possible extension of my life in making decisions concerning life-sustaining treatment.

I want my life to be prolonged and I want life-sustaining treatment to be provided unless I am in a coma or persistent vegetative state that my doctor reasonably believes to be irreversible. Once my doctor has reasonably concluded that I will remain unconscious for the rest of my life, I do not want life-sustaining treatment to be provided or continued.

I want my life to be prolonged to the greatest extent possible without regard to my condition, the chances I have for recovery or the cost of the procedures.

Some charities provide forms on which you can write out any specific wishes. You are not required to give specific details but may wish to do so.

Knowing what details to write is complicated because none of us knows the exact circumstances in which it will be acted on. However, you can get some idea by asking your doctor about what they think might be the most likely developments for someone with your condition. Your specific instructions can discuss outcomes, particular circumstances, or both. If you discuss outcomes, then the statement should focus on what types of outcomes would be acceptable and which would not. For example, "resuscitate if my mental functions will be unimpaired."

It is an important self-management task to find out about possible circumstances arising from your particular condition. Consider how much treatment you would want to be given, for example, if you developed pneumonia, or if your heart stopped. Would you wish to be fed through a tube? Would you wish to have mechanical ventilation to help with breathing, if problems arose with that? Think about the circumstances in which you would have a particular wish.

Getting Your Wishes Carried Out

So you have done the difficult personal exploration of your feelings, and you have sorted out what you want. Many people get this far. That is, they have thought through their wishes about dying and have even written them down in a living will. This is an excellent beginning, but not the end of the job. A good self-manager has to do more than just write a note. They have to see that it gets acted on. If you really want your wishes carried out, it is important that you share them fully with your family, your doctor and anyone you wish to act for you. This is often not an easy task. The following section discusses ways to make these conversations easier.

Before you can have a conversation, it is a good idea for all interested parties to be aware of your living will. If your living will specifies refusal of life-saving treatments remember that it is necessary to have it signed and witnessed. Make several copies. You may need copies for family members, your doctor and other interested parties. It may also be helpful to give one to your solicitor.

Now you are ready to talk about your wishes. You may find that those you need to talk to, have some difficulty discussing death with you. Few people find it easy to discuss their own death or that of a loved one. So, you may receive the response, "Oh, don't think about that", or "That's a long time off", or "Don't be so morbid, you're not that ill." Unfortunately, this is usually enough to end the conversation. Your job as a good self-manager is to keep the conversation open. There are several ways to do this.

Plan how you will begin your discussion of this subject. Here are some suggestions.

Prepare your living will, and then give copies to the appropriate family members or friends. Ask them to read it and then set a specific time to discuss it. If they respond as in the examples above, say that you understand this is a difficult topic, but that it's important to you to discuss it with them. This is a good time to practise the 'I' messages discussed in chapter 9. For example, "I understand that death is a difficult thing to talk about. However, it is very important to me that we have this discussion."

You might suggest that everybody in your family makes a living will and then shares them. Present this as an important aspect of being a mature adult and family member. Making this a family project in which everyone is involved may make it easier to discuss. In addition, it would help to clarify everyone's values about the topics of death and dying.

Write a letter or an email, or prepare a video or CD which can be sent to members of your family. State that you feel your death is an important topic to discuss and that you want them to know your wishes. Then state your wishes, providing reasons for the choices you indicate. At the same time, send them a copy of your living will. Importantly, at this point ask them to respond in some way or to arrange with you to set aside some time to talk in person or on the phone.

Talking to Your Doctor

It can be hard to talk to your doctor, too, about your wishes surrounding death. In fact, only a very small percentage of people who have living wills ever share them with their doctor.

There are several reasons why it's important to do this. First, you need to be sure your doctor is aware of your values. If you and your doctor don't have the same values, it may be difficult for them to understand your wishes. Second, your doctor needs to know what you want. It is important to give your doctor a copy of your living will so that it can become a permanent part of your medical record.

Perhaps make an appointment with your doctor to discuss the issues. This should not be a quick word at the end of a regular visit. Rather, say at the beginning, "May I have a few minutes to discuss with you my wishes in the event of a serious problem or impending death." Most doctors will make time to talk to you. If the doctor says there is not enough time, then ask to make another appointment. This is a situation in which you may need to be assertive. Doctors may find this a difficult topic to discuss with their patients. After all, they are in the business of helping to keep people alive and well. They don't like to think about their patients dying. On the other hand, most doctors want their patients to have Lasting Powers of Attorney for health care, because this relieves them of pressure and worry. They might say, "Oh, you don't have to worry about that, let me do it," or "We'll worry about that when the time comes." Using an "I" message, as in chapter 9, to communicate that this is important to you might help you assert yourself if this happens. Doctors don't want to worry you and may think they are doing you a favour by not describing everything that might happen or the treatment options. You can help by telling your doctor that having control and making some decisions about your future will ease your mind. Not knowing or not being clear on what could happen is more worrying than being faced with the facts and dealing with them.

You might want to bring someone with you when you see the doctor. A third person present can make it easier to talk and, at the same time, they can meet your doctor. This provides an opportunity to clarify any misunderstandings about your wishes. It opens the lines of communication between your family and doctor. At the very least, post your doctor a copy of your living will to be placed in your medical records.

When you go to hospital, be sure the hospital has a copy of the living will. Don't put it in your safe deposit box—no one will be able to get it when it is needed.

Keeping Your Documents Up To Date

Now you have done all the important things. The hard work is over. However, remember that you can change your mind at any time. The person you want to act for you might no longer be available or your wishes might change. Be sure to keep these documents updated. Like any legal document, it can be revoked or changed at any time. The decisions you make today are not forever

Making your wishes known about how you want to be treated in case of serious or life-threatening illness is one of the most important tasks of self-management. The best way to do this is to prepare a living will and share this with your family, close friends, and doctor.

A Few More Notes About Preparing for Death and Seeking Hospice Care

In most parts of the country hospice care is available. In everyone's life there comes a time when medical care is no longer helpful and we need to prepare for death. Today, we often have several weeks or months to make these preparations. This is when hospice care is so very useful. The aim of hospice care is to provide a terminally ill patient with the highest quality of life possible. At the same time, hospice professionals help the patient and family prepare for death with dignity, and help the surviving family members. Some people choose hospice "home support" programmes. This means that the patient stays in their own home and the services come to them. In some places there are also residential hospices where people can go for their last days.

Sometimes people wait until the last few days before death to ask for hospice care. They somehow see it as "giving up." However, they may put an unnecessary burden on themselves, friends and family. The reverse may also be true. Families wish to look after a sick person without help. Everybody concerned might consider whether the patient's life and dying could be better if a hospice cares for all the medical things so that family and friends are free to give love and support.

Most hospices only accept people who are expected to die within six months. This does not mean people are thrown out if they "outlive" their time. Six months is a guideline, not a fixed time. If you, a family member or a friend is in the last stage of illness, find and make use of your local hospice. It is a wonderful final gift.

Making your wishes known in a living will is an important part of self-management. Like other self-management tasks, some hard work now can reward you with improved quality of life.

• • •

Suggested Further Reading

Cantor, Norman L. *Advance Directives and the Pursuit of Death With Dignity*. Bloomington, Ind.: Indiana University Press, 1993.

Elkington, J., and Hailes, J. *Manual 2000: Life Choices for the Future You Want*. Hodder and Stoughton, 1998.

Emanuel, Linda. "How Living Wills Can Help Doctors and Patients Talk About Dying: They Can Open the Door to a Positive, Caring Approach to Death." *British Medical Journal*, 320 (7250), pp. 1618-19, 17 June 2000. Discusses how living wills can be used positively to help prepare for death.

Molloy, W., and Mepham, V. *Let Me Decide: The Health Care Directive That Speaks for You When You Can't*. Penguin, 1993.

Patients Association, British Medical Association. *Advance Statements About Future Medical Treatment: A Guide for Patients*. Patients Association, 1997.

Other Resources

Some good websites with information are www.ageconcern.co.uk, www.alzheimers.org.uk, www.growthhouse.org and http://www.direct.gov.uk/en/RightsAndResponsibilities/Death/index.htm

Office of Public Guardianship
Archway Tower
2 Junction Road
London N19 5SZ
Document Exchange: DX 141150 Archway 2
Email: custserv@guardianship.gsi.gov.uk (the email and web address are to change)
Website: www.guardianship.gov.uk/

NB: The Court of Protection is also at this address

General Contact Numbers
Customer Literature and Application Forms
9am–6pm, Mon–Fri
Tel: 0845 330 2900 (local call rate)
Fax: 0870 739 5780 (UK callers)
or +44 207 664 7000 (for callers outside UK)

Text Phone
9am–5pm, Mon–Fri
Tel: 020 7664 7755
If you have speech or hearing difficulties, and you have access to a text phone, you can call the OPG text phone and a customer service operator will assist you.

Legal information is correct as of June 2007 and should not be used as a substitute for getting fuller appropriate legal advice.

EPP CIC thanks Solicitors for the Elderly for legal checking of this chapter.

Solicitors for the Elderly public contact telephone:
01992 471568

Post contact details:
Solicitors for the Elderly Ltd
Room 17
Conbar House
Mead Lane
Hertford
Herts
SG13 7AP

CHAPTER
12

Healthy Eating

There is an enormous amount of information available to us about food and drink. Books, newspapers, television, radio, the Internet, magazines—these reflect the interest everyone feels in health and in food, as well as fashion and appearance. There is a constant stream from the media of more or less reliable, sometimes contradictory information, until we hardly know who to believe. Luckily, as an active self-manager, you are uniquely placed to assess how you feel when you eat and drink in a particular way and can make your own healthy decisions.

The self-management task around food is, as with other aspects of a healthy life, to review this aspect of your situation. Find good information from reliable sources, decide what—if anything—you want to change in your current way of eating, work out how to try the changes for yourself, do it and assess the results.

Reviewing and changing involves feelings, of course. You may find yourself having to explore feelings which seem at first unrelated to food. Because of the need for gathering information and reflecting on it, you may find that the action planning and problem-solving approach from chapter 2 will adapt itself very well to this aspect of your life.

In particular, the journal or calendar suggested for use in relation to symptom management and in working out an appropriate exercise programme may well come in useful for recording some notes about what you eat. There is a sample "food-mood" diary sheet on page 204. If you are clear about what actually (honestly!) goes into your mouth, you will be able to evaluate any small changes you make. When you feel better, you will be well-placed to continue your improvements. You will, as in other areas of self-management, be rewarded by beginning to take to control of what you eat and drink.

Developing healthy eating habits is important for everyone. We know that eating nutritious food gives us energy and endurance, and it makes us feel better physically and emotionally. It reduces the risk of certain health problems. The effects of a particular way of eating can also be an aspect of symptom management, and reviewing your food intake might be a way into the circle of tangled symptoms as discussed in chapter 2. While food alone cannot prevent or cure a chronic condition, learning to make healthier choices in the foods we eat can help us manage symptoms, prevent complications, and feel more in control of our health.

Start your review with a look at your first-stage food-processing tools—your teeth. Anyone who has ever had toothache, or a broken tooth, or uncomfortable dentures, or an insecure crown will know how miserably difficult it is to chew properly, let alone enjoy food, if there is discomfort in your mouth. Make your dentist your friend as well as one of your professional consultants. Keep on going until your problem is sorted out.

Problems around chewing may centre on a dry mouth. Drinking water half an hour before you eat may make that easier, and we all benefit from keeping ourselves properly hydrated.

If you have had surgical intervention or some treatment around your nose, throat or mouth, which affects your chewing, your swallowing or your sense of smell or taste, take that into account in your review of your diet. Consult your practitioners to make sure you are comfortable as you can possibly be and make it a goal to devise ways of making your food manageable and palatable.

What is Healthy Eating?—The Balance of Good Health

This chapter suggests that you look at the "balance" of the food you eat. Most of us eat fairly well a lot of the time, but a review of our eating habits may show up areas we can improve, especially in relation to a long-term condition. It suggests that achieving balance may require only a few, easy changes. It offers you some suggestions on how you might begin making small changes in your eating habits to bring balance by reducing or leaving out some foods and adding others. It includes tips for planning well-balanced meals, making healthier food choices, managing a healthy weight, and for minimising some of the problems commonly associated with eating and weight management.

Take Small Steps

You can't change everything all at once. You probably don't need to. But anyway it may not be sensible even to try. What we eat and how we prepare it are habits that have developed over a lifetime. Eating is an important part of all our lives and part of healthy eating is enjoying it. We choose particular foods for all sorts of reasons, not just to get calories and nutrients, but because of its taste, smell, colour, and appearance. We are also influenced by cost and availability. Living in society means we take on cultural influences too. Sharing meals is one of the ways we relate to family and friends. It's how we show and accept love and hospitality. For many of us, meals are an important part of our religious practice. Healthy eating isn't just about refuelling ourselves, like putting petrol in a car! So changes in our diet need thought and care. Suddenly trying to change everything about the way we eat is unrealistic. The fact is that small changes which are well-informed, clearly decided, consciously carried out and properly reviewed, are more likely to be sustained, and can make noticeable and relatively rapid changes in our health.

What we do routinely, every day, around food, is what needs review. The occasional indulgence in a little of what we fancy isn't usually a problem, providing there is a solid supply of nutritious food regularly available to our bodies. We would all probably accept that some choices of food can improve how we feel in the longer term. The notion of balance applies to choosing the larger part of what we eat with an eye to providing ourselves with all the basics for repair and healing, in the proportions that our bodies can use most efficiently. So it's sensible to take note of what both research and individual experience have found—that balancing our nutrition by eating less fat, sugar, salt, refined and processed foods, and more starchy, unrefined foods, fruit and vegetables makes us function, and feel, better. Moderating our intake of tea, coffee, sweet soft drinks and alcohol shifts the balance of our drinking to allow us more water, needed by our bodies for maintaining good health. There may be specific dietary requirements for your long-term condition, which obviously you will take into account, but as a general principle, healthy eating for all of us requires balancing our overall intake and reviewing it periodically, to get the best we can out of what we eat.

A well-balanced meal or snack might include:

- One portion of protein-rich foods, meat or fish or alternatives, making up a quarter of your meal
- One or more portions of vegetables, not counting potatoes, making up at least half your meal
- One portion of carbohydrate-rich wholegrain products like pasta, and one of vegetables that are high in starch, maybe potatoes, making up the other quarter of your meal
- One portion of fruit or fruit juice

Tips for Healthy Eating

- Enjoy your food.
- Chew it thoroughly!
- Eat a variety of good-quality foods.
- Eat very little fat.
- Eat plenty of foods rich in starch and fibre.
- Eat plenty of fresh fruit and fresh vegetables.
- Eat very little sugar.
- Eat very little salt.
- Eat regularly and in moderation.
- Eat the right amount to be a healthy weight.
- Limit tea, coffee and soft drinks.
- Drink very little alcohol.
- Drink water.
- Take note of what your doctor says about the right food for your condition.
- Have a look now and again at the effect on you of what you are eating, and be prepared to change.

Find Your Balance

To eat healthily, in a balanced way, follow these basic principles.

Eat a wide variety of foods, eat regular meals at the same times every day, and try to eat the same amount of food at each meal.

Eating a variety of foods is important so that the body gets all the essential nutrients it needs to function well. Our body takes nutrients from the items of food we choose by the process of digestion—that is, it breaks down the food chemically during chewing, passing it through the stomach and through the intestines which extract usable nutritious substances and discard the rest. The nutrients we

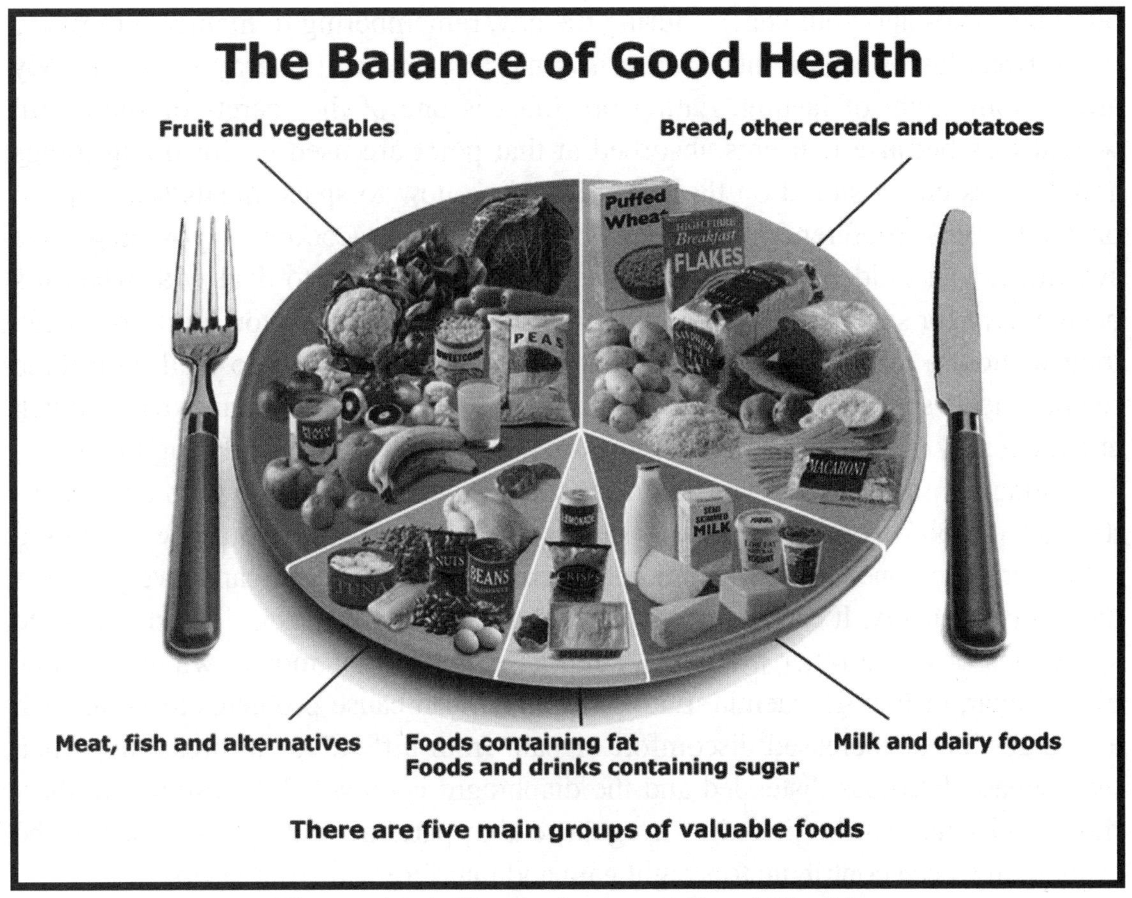

Figure 12.1 *The Balance of Good Health*

need are proteins, carbohydrates, fat, vitamins, and minerals. Each plays an important role and can be found in varying amounts in the different food groups. "Food groups" is a way of classifying what we eat to give us some basic, "balancing" information about what we choose. Since measuring nutrients is not an exact science, choosing a balanced variety of foods is a way of covering our bases—over a period of a week or two, we will be providing our body with what it needs. Taking vitamins and food supplements can never replace eating a variety of foods. These "extras" contain only the nutrients we know about. To get all essential nutrients, both known and unknown, we need to eat a good assortment of the foods available to us. Apart from anything else, eating the same foods too often can be dull, and choosing as wide a variety as is possible in our situation can be a source of interest and pleasure—both healthy aims!

Eating something when you get up in the morning every day, and then eating regularly throughout the day, provides the body with the fuel it needs to function well all the time. It keeps you feeling energetic. For this reason, it is best to space out your meals and your snacks during the day, remembering to include a morning meal. Breakfast is important because it is the first boost of energy for your body after a long night of fasting. Eating breakfast is one of the secrets of successful weight loss because nutrients absorbed at that point are used up for doing things and are less easily stored on the body. Deciding how to space meals will depend on your needs, preferences, and lifestyle, but do take account of your digestive system. If you suddenly hit it with a huge amount of food to deal with when it's been empty for several hours, it is likely to protest—as it is if you let it go for too long without a job to do. Listen to your insides. Some people do well with three regular meals spaced four to five hours apart, while others who cannot eat as much at a meal may need to eat smaller, more frequent meals or snacks during the day.

Eating the same amount at each meal respects your digestive system and allows it to do its job of providing a consistent supply of energy for our use. Skipping meals, or eating one large meal and not much the rest of the day, can leave you with dips in your energy. It can lead to unplanned and unhealthy snacks. It can aggravate symptoms or cause other problems, such as irritability or mood swings and low blood sugar, or hypoglycaemia. Eating too much can cause problems as well, such as indigestion or increased discomfort or pain from difficulties in breathing, when the stomach becomes distended and the diaphragm is crowded. Constipation, diarrhoea and wind can be linked to irregular eating patterns. Eating too much at the evening meal can contribute to weight gain and interfere with your sleep.

Now, you are probably asking yourself, "What is the right amount to eat at each meal?" Unfortunately, there is no one simple or right answer to this question for everyone. You are your own best guide in this area. You will know if you regularly feel uncomfortable after a particular food, or if you have eaten too much, or if you have patches when your energy drops. These are matters for careful review in your food diary. If you find you can't solve them, you may wish to look for, or ask one of your consultants about, information on recommended portion sizes or overall quantities.

Know Your Food Groups

Bread, Other Cereals, and Potatoes

Starchy foods should form the main part of your meals, because carbohydrate provides much of the energy we need for movement and warmth. This group includes bread, rolls, chapattis, breakfast cereals, oats, pasta, noodles, rice, potatoes, sweet potatoes, plantains and green bananas, beans and lentils, and dishes made from maize, millet, barley and cornmeal, but not potato crisps, because they are so high in fat and salt that they are not balanced. Potatoes are, of course, vegetables, but because they are so starchy they appear in this group. These foods only contribute to balance if you don't cover them with butter, oil or salt when you eat them!

The wholegrain varieties of starchy foods not only provide sustained energy over several hours but are also a good source of fibre, which our bodies need for healthy guts. We need a substantial proportion of wholemeal bread, brown rice, or wholegrain pasta in our daily intake. Baked beans are also a quick, cheap and tasty source of fibre.

Fruit and Vegetables

Eat at least five portions of fruit and vegetables each day, the fresher the better. One portion is about a medium sized apple or banana, a bowl of salad or two tablespoonfuls of vegetables or beans. This group includes vegetables and salad as well as all fresh, frozen and canned fruit, though choose the ones in natural juice. Beans and lentils, dried fruit and a glass of fruit juice can also contribute to fruit and vegetable intake but keep up the variety—five glasses of juice a day won't do the trick! Potatoes and nuts are not included in this group. Choosing a wide variety from this group helps to ensure you are getting all the vitamins and minerals you need.

Milk and Dairy Foods

This group includes milk, cheese, yoghurt and fromage frais. Butter is also dairy but is listed in the "fats" group because it is so high in fats. Dairy foods can all be high in fat, particularly saturated fat, which is the kind of fat that does not promote health, so choose lower or reduced fat versions whenever possible. Most people use cow's milk, but investigate goat's, sheep's and soya milk or oat milk or rice milk which can provide a suitable, digestible alternative for some people and may also tip the balance if you need to.

Meat, Fish, and Alternative Sources of Protein

This group includes lamb, pork and beef, known as red meats, white meat such as chicken and turkey, and fish, including white fish, such as cod and haddock, and oily fish, such as salmon, herring, mackerel and tuna. Alternatives to meat and fish, such as eggs, beans and pulses, nuts and nut products, such as peanut butter, textured vegetable protein and tofu—all these provide protein. Once again, for balance, use your judgment about the nutrients within any one choice of food—use lean meat , cutting off any visible fat, and be wary of meat and fish products, that is, sausages, pies, meatballs, fish fingers and fish cakes which can contain very high levels of fat, salt, sugar and preservative—check the labels. "Oily" fish, however, such as tinned or fresh sardines, mackerel or salmon gives you the sort of fat that is necessary for health and you can eat that once or twice a week.

Fats, Oils and Sugar

These appear often in foods that can help to add taste, variety and enjoyment to the diet. There is no need to avoid them totally, but it is best to limit your intake. A small amount of fat is essential for health, but most of us eat more than we need.

Foods containing fat include butter, margarine, low-fat spreads, cooking oils, mayonnaise and salad dressings. Use these foods sparingly and choose lower or reduced fat versions when possible.

Foods containing sugar include biscuits, cakes, puddings, ice-cream, chocolate, sweets, crisps, sugar, and sugar sweetened drinks. Don't have these often and when you do, have small amounts.

Fibre—An Extra, But Not Optional

Fibre doesn't quite fit into a food group, but is essential for healthy eating. During the process of digestion, food moves steadily through you, with all the useful nutrients gradually extracted. The muscular activity to keep things moving from top to bottom is much helped by the right sort of fibrous bulk, which will be discarded at the end of the process. If you eat very refined food, with no fibrous husks or vegetable fibre left in it, your body will have trouble shifting the unusable or toxic matter. Therefore, waste may stay in your system longer than is healthy, and that produces uncomfortable symptoms of its own.

Water—The Forgotten Facilitator

Also not in a food group, but in lots of food, and a major component of our body. Extracting and using the nutrients in our food depends on having enough water passing through us, as well as the food. Cells absorb nutrients dissolved in water. It is a large part of our blood. With fibre, it is essential to the proper progress of food, and waste, through our gut. It aids elimination and keeps the kidneys functioning properly. Drinking enough water helps you to eat less. Incidentally it also helps prevent medication side-effects.

Know Your Nutrients

From the different food groups, our body extracts what it needs. The body doesn't recognise which actual foods it's getting. We do that part of the choosing when we decide what to put in our mouths. After that, the digestive system takes over, starting with teeth, tongue and saliva. The body breaks all our food down into various nutrients which it metabolises to keep us warm, alive and well. These nutrients are protein, carbohydrates, fats, vitamins and minerals.

Proteins are made from amino acids, the basic chemical "building blocks" of life. Digestion breaks the proteins down so our body can use them to make enzymes and hormones, to maintain the immune system, to fight infection and to build or repair damaged tissues. Our body makes some of its energy from protein. Meat, fish, poultry, eggs, and dairy products provide complete proteins—that is, all the amino acids are present. Vegetable proteins such as those in legumes, grains, nuts, and seeds can be incomplete but when you eat them in the right combinations in the same meal, like rice with lentils or beans on toast, complete proteins become available. Vegetable proteins are good value nutritionally because they are low in fat, high in fibre and contain no cholesterol.

The second nutrient to look at is carbohydrate, which our digestive system extracts and uses as the major source of energy for our bodily processes. The heat that any one food can produce in our body is what we measure in calories. We need to eat a high proportion of food containing carbohydrates each day to keep steady our basic body temperature and our energy to move around. Starches, or complex carbohydrates, occur in grains, rice, pasta, breads, peas and beans, root vegetables such as potatoes and carrots, and other vegetables. Complex carbohydrates take time to digest and so they help keep blood sugar levels constant, which we want. Simple carbohydrates, or sugars, are found in fruits and some dairy products. These are good sources of carbohydrate, which are very quickly absorbed, but in terms of the balance of our intake they need watching, especially processed foods that are made with refined or table sugar, honey, syrups, and jellies. These forms of simple carbohydrate do very little good to balance the calories they provide, and have the added disadvantage of sending blood sugar levels up very fast and letting them drop again, which we don't want. Incidentally, grains and vegetables also provide an excellent source of fibre.

The third nutrient our body needs is a very small amount of "good" fat. Fats are fatty acids bound together with glycerol. Fats can be saturated, which we do not need, mono-unsaturated, or polyunsaturated which are "good". Our bodies use fat for energy. We also need it to build, strengthen and repair tissues. But if we eat more than we need in a day, we store the rest. That sends our weight up. Excess stored fat has been linked to various health risks. You get lots of fat from meat, whole-milk dairy products, nuts, seeds, peanuts, and oils. Fat provides twice as many calories per gram as proteins or carbohydrates, so it's better to limit the amount of fat you eat, especially the saturated fats from animal sources and processed foods. Limiting foods that are high in saturated fat also helps to reduce the cholesterol we get from our diets. Cholesterol is not a fat but tends to be present in high-fat dairy products, meats, and poultry.

Finally, our body also needs small amounts—traces, sometimes, too small to be measured—of many vitamins and minerals, for a large number of vital functions. Vitamins and minerals are found in varying amounts in different foods, depending on how and where the food was produced. That's one reason why we need to eat a variety of fresh, good quality foods, grown in good, healthy soil.

Some people may benefit from supplements, not to take the place of a balanced choice of foodstuffs, but to help reach the recommended daily allowance of a particular vitamin or mineral. However, you can waste a lot of money on supplements if you don't find out all you can about what to take, and it may save trouble and expense to add a nutritional or dietary practitioner to your network of consultants. Too much of some vitamins or minerals can create health problems and even some toxic reactions, and too little can make you think that something potentially helpful has made no difference.

Balance Your Diet

Eat More Starchy Foods and Fibre

For most people, the move towards a healthier diet will mean eating more starchy foods. Starchy foods are low in fat and help to fill you up, particularly "wholegrain" or "high fibre" varieties.

- Build your meals around vegetables, whole-grain products, and fruits.
- Eat a variety of fruits and vegetables, raw or slightly cooked.
- Eat whole fruit rather than drinking fruit juice.
- Eat low-fat grain products such as whole-wheat breads, brown rice, and corn tortillas instead of white flour pastas, white flour tortillas and white rice.
- Eat foods made with oats, barley, corn, dried beans, peas and lentils at least a few times each week and as meat substitutes.
- Choose shredded wheat, grape nuts, or raisin bran for cold breakfast cereals.
- Eat higher-fibre crispbread, such as whole-rye or multigrain crackers, with sesame or pumpkin or sunflower seeds.
- Choose foods with whole wheat or whole grain listed as the first ingredient.
- Add fibre gradually over a period of a few weeks and drink plenty of water to help move the fibre through your system.
- Simply, increase the amount of, say, pasta, that you serve, so it makes up a larger proportion of the food on the plate.

Eat Less Fat

A small amount of fat in the diet is essential for our health, but most of us eat far too much. Some fats are easy to spot like cream, the fat on the outside of meat, butter and margarine. There are also "hidden" fats in cakes, chocolate, biscuits, crisps, mayonnaise and pastry so for these you have to read the labels.

- Weigh out, say, ten grams of butter so you can visualise how much fat is in anything you eat.
- Choose lower or reduced fat spreads, and spread them more thinly.
- Reduce or, sometimes, cut out spread, for example with beans on toast.

- Use semi-skimmed or skimmed milk.
- Use low-fat yoghurt or low-fat fromage frais instead of cream.
- Choose half-fat hard cheese or cottage cheese, or use a small amount of a very strong cheese, such as parmesan.
- Make salad dressings with natural yoghurt, herbs, spices, tomato juice, vinegar or lemon instead.
- Cut out crisps, chocolates, cakes, pastries and biscuits.
- Remove the skin from chicken, duck and turkey before cooking.
- Eat more poultry—chicken, turkey, eat less red meat—beef, lamb, venison, mutton, pork
- Grill, microwave, steam, poach, bake or boil food rather than roasting or frying.
- Use a good-quality non-stick pan with a cooking oil spray.
- Avoid deep-fried food.
- Skim fat off soups and stews—cool, refrigerate and remove solidified fat from casseroles and stews. This generally improves the flavour as well. When you re-heat, take the temperature to boiling point and then simmer for a couple of minutes.
- Buy the leanest cuts of meat you can afford and trim off all the visible fat.
- Choose low fat versions of sausages and other meat products.
- Use as little oil, margarine or butter for cooking as possible—choose baked or boiled potatoes rather than chips or roast.
- Choose lower fat sauces, tomato-based perhaps, to eat with rice and pasta. You can also change the amounts served—a little less sauce and a little more pasta.

Eat Less Sugar

Eating a lot of sugar can cause tooth decay. It can also make you fat, without providing any nutrition at all.

- Try tea and coffee without sugar. Cut down a little at a time. If you really can't give it up, try using one of the artificial sweeteners.
- Keep soft drinks for treats. They are very high in sugar and often contain colouring and preservatives which your body does not need. Drink tap-water—filtering it often improves the taste—or bottled still water.
- Read breakfast cereal packets to find exactly how much hidden sugar you will be eating. Use fresh, dried or canned fruit to sweeten breakfast cereals, cakes or puddings rather than using sugar. Choose wholegrain breakfast cereals rather than those coated with sugar or honey.
- Buy fruit canned in natural, unsweetened juice rather than in syrup.
- Go easy on cakes, biscuits, pastries, sweets and chocolate.
- Cut down on jam, marmalade, syrup, treacle and honey.
- Use low-sugar varieties of any ready-made puddings and desserts you buy.
- Dried fruits contain high concentrations of sugar and can become stuck around the teeth, so avoid eating them frequently between meals.

Eat Less Salt

Salt is the main source of sodium in the diet. Most of us have more sodium in our diets than we need.

- Don't add salt during cooking.
- Don't add salt to food at the table and certainly not until you have tasted it. Flavour foods with lemon juice, herbs, spices, or cider vinegar instead of salt.

- Cut out salty snack foods like crisps, salted nuts and other salty nibbles.
- If you buy canned vegetables, choose the ones labelled 'no added salt'.
- Don't eat salted meat such as bacon, gammon and salt beef very often.
- Stock cubes are very salty. Try making your own stock or using fewer stock cubes but adding more herbs, garlic and spices for flavour.
- Many ready-prepared savoury dishes and sauces are very salty. Look at the label to find those with less added salt—sodium—and monosodium glutamate.
- Biscuits, breakfast cereals and pre-cooked foods tend to have hidden salt—check the ingredients on the label.
- Limit sauces high in salt such as soy sauce.
- Salt substitutes can help reduce the amount of sodium in the diet—particularly if you miss the taste of salt. However, most salt substitutes still contain some salt. So, if you really want to lose the taste for salt, it is best to cut it out bit by bit, so you gradually learn to taste the food itself again.
- Check the sodium levels of the bottled water you buy. Read labels to compare brands and choose the lowest number.
- There is little difference between sea salt and normal salt. As sea salt is often sold as crystals, you might end up eating more salt than you would use normal table salt.

Improve Your Balance

The Balance of Good Health (Figure 12.1) stresses that a healthy diet is one based on wide variety, with plenty of starchy foods, plus fruit and vegetables. A healthy diet also means enjoying the food you eat and not skipping meals, such as breakfast. Everything you eat, snacks, half-biscuits and all, counts towards the balance of your diet. Many of the dishes we eat are a combination of foods from several of the food groups—like casseroles, spaghetti bolognaise, sandwiches and pizza. To make a healthier choice, it is important to think about how the main ingredients of any dish fit with the proportions shown in the Balance of Good Health. We don't always eat at home, or we don't cook from scratch, or we are in a hurry, or we eat out, so we need to think about improving the balance of the meals we are not completely in charge of.

Here are some small changes towards practising healthy eating, whether you are eating at home, at work, in a café or at a restaurant, by balancing the available choices.

Balance Your Breakfast

If your breakfast has been porridge and coffee, use skim milk for them both. Add fresh or dried fruit. If it's normally cornflakes, use wholegrain, wholewheat or "high fibre" version, with skim milk. Add oat bran or wheat bran to your normal cereal to increase fibre. If you use sugar on your cereal, try soaked raisins instead, or chop a banana on top. If you go for white toast, start making it from wholewheat bread, use low-fat vegetable spread instead of butter and go easy on the marmalade. Have a glass of fresh fruit juice.

Balance Your Snacks

Eat:

- Fresh fruit
- Vegetable based soups
- Pizza made on bread rolls or scone base with vegetables and a little half-fat hard cheese
- Sardines or baked beans on toast
- Wholegrain breakfast cereals, not coated with sugar or honey, served with skimmed or semi-skimmed milk or eaten straight from the packet
- Plain popcorn sprinkled with paprika or Parmesan cheese
- Bread sticks, wholegrain crackers, crispbreads or rice-cakes with low-fat toppings—a scrape of tahini or a nut butter
- Unsalted nuts

Balance Eating Out and Take-Aways

Restaurant, cafe, and take-away meals are often convenient and tasty, but can be high in fat. You may be able to ask for your meal or snack to be prepared with less fat and more vegetables—ask when you order. Vegetarian options may not be automatically healthier if they are cooked with a lot of oil, cream or cheese.

Choose:

- Sandwiches with lower fat fillings
- Salads without dressing or with lower fat dressing, for example, yoghurt dressing
- Baked potato without butter and with low-fat fillings such as cottage cheese, baked beans, ratatouille, chicken and mushroom, tuna without mayonnaise or chilli con carne
- Burgers made of beef, chicken, fish or bean, in wholemeal buns with salad—skip the cheese and mayonnaise
- Meat, fish or pasta without creamy sauces
- Shish kebabs in pitta bread with salad which are a healthier option than doner kebabs
- Large helping of plain noodles or rice with stir-fried vegetables
- Tandoori chicken or chicken tikka with salad and chapattis or rice
- A pizza, with less cheese but extra vegetables
- Vegetables or salad with your meal instead of chips

Balance Your Lunch

You can make small changes to the main meals you cook, and have a big effect on the balance of your overall intake.

Review your recipes:

- For spaghetti bolognaise with mincemeat, cooked with onion, carrots, celery, herbs, spices, tomato paste and tinned tomatoes, served with pasta, use lean mince or skim the fat during cooking, add more vegetables to the sauce than you have habitually done — such as extra tinned tomatoes and peppers. Increase the serving of pasta and decrease the amount of sauce. Add a side salad. You barely notice the difference but your body has more of what it needs.

- For a roast meal, of chicken, potatoes, carrots and gravy, reduce the fat content by skinning the chicken before you cook it, by replacing the roast potatoes with jacket or boiled, and skimming off the fat from the pan juice before you make gravy. Add an extra vegetable, and the meal is higher in fibre and lower in fat, better balanced and healthier.

- A vegetable lasagne might start with plenty of vegetables cooked in a minimum of oil, a white sauce made with cornflour and skimmed milk, half-fat cheese or a small amount of Parmesan, plus extra vegetables or a side salad. A bread roll can fill any gaps without sending up the fat intake—and your meal is more healthily balanced.
- A meal of fish fingers, mashed potatoes, frozen mixed vegetables doesn't need butter in the potatoes, use some chopped herbs instead. Grill or bake the fish fingers rather than frying them. Serve more vegetables than you have done in the past.

Balance Your Packed Lunch

Thinking of interesting and tasty packed lunches every day taxes anyone's imagination, but with a stock of bread and a variety of fresh vegetables in the fridge you can produce tasty and attractive portable meals, well-balanced nutritionally.

- Make sandwiches with thick-cut wholemeal bread, wholewheat rolls, crispbreads which can also be made of grains other than wheat, muffins, chapattis, wraps and pitta breads provide variety and increase nutritional value.
- Use a low-fat spread or replace with nut butter or low-fat cream cheese.
- Use fillings such as lean meat, chicken, boiled egg, mashed banana, low-fat cottage cheese, half-fat hard cheese, tuna, sardines, chopped raw vegetables, bean and nut spreads.

- Take pasta or rice salad instead of sandwiches—for example, wholewheat pasta shells or pasta made of buckwheat or cornmeal plus pepper, cucumber chunks, cold chopped chicken, tuna or kidney beans—these provide a nutritionally well-balanced mixture of food types. You can use lemon juice or cider vinegar to add flavour—both these contain useful vitamins and minerals.
- Raw vegetables such as baby tomatoes or sticks of carrot and cucumber or cauliflower florets with a hummus or taramasalata dip.
- Soup, baked beans or pasta in sauce, in a wide-necked thermos flask with bread
- Currant buns without icing, scones or teabreads
- Low-fat yoghurt or low-fat fromage frais
- Fresh fruit, such as apples, oranges, pears or peaches
- Dried fruit such as apricots or raisins

Balance Your Ready Meals

- Read the labels. Select those that are lower in fat, sugar and salt. Most supermarkets now sell pre-prepared meals that are labelled as being healthier options, but you still need to read the labels to make sure they suit you—some "low-fat" biscuits, for example, are higher in sugar.
- Add vegetables to the meal—if convenient or necessary use pre-washed, frozen or canned. Serve more than you have usually done in the past and you will improve the balance of your meal.
- Serve wholemeal bread or pitta, whole brown rice, potatoes, or wholewheat pasta with the meal. These gently increase your carbohydrate and fibre intake.
- Fruit, low-fat yoghurt or low-fat fromage frais are quick, ready-prepared desserts.

- Some common meals—beans on toast, vegetable based soups, microwaved baked potatoes—are healthy options which are as quick or quicker to prepare and cook than many ready-made meals.

Balance Your Puddings

You don't need to say goodbye to puddings and desserts. Fruit, fresh, dried or tinned in juice, not syrup, makes an excellent alternative to pudding. You can also add fruit to rice pudding or custard, made with low fat milk. If you are making your own cakes or puddings, use lower fat ingredients, skimmed milk rather than whole, low-fat yoghurt or fromage frais instead of cream, dried fruit instead of sugar.

Check Food Labels

You need to know what you are eating in detail before you can think about balancing it.

Most of us have eaten foods that come from a can, box, package, or some other type of container. With the exception of foods prepared in the shop or some of those from small manufacturers, most food packages are required to provide nutritional information, unless the package is too small to list it all. In this case, the manufacturer usually includes a telephone number or address for you to contact them.

A lot of information appears in very small print on food labels. Part of your information–gathering when you review your eating pattern will be to tackle labels. Take your time and your specs! Many food labels list the amount of calories and fat in the food. Probably your main interest at the start is to check for calories, sugar, salt and fat. Your aim will be to make the healthier choice from amongst the available options—as you get more practised, you could find that you move away from packaged food to those which are less complicated and less processed. Anyway, you will often find there is a useful difference between two brands, enough to make the small changes you are looking for.

Some food labels make claims that the food has particular benefits. Specific claims like "low in calories" or "rich in vitamin C" have to meet legal conditions. Vague claims like "natural goodness" are meaningless from a health point of view. Many manufacturers and supermarkets use labels or symbols to identify foods that are lower in fat, sugar or salt, or higher in fibre. These can be useful as a quick guide, but if you are concerned about the content of foods, it is best to compare the food labels in detail. When a claim such as 'low-fat' is made, it is compulsory to give nutritional information on the label. "Lower" fat suggests that something else is "higher", not that it is automatically "good for you". Use the '100g' column to compare different products of similar kinds of foods and to choose the lower fat, sugar and salt sodium varieties.

Food Additives

Additives are added to packaged food to help prolong its storage life, to make it easier to manufacture, to improve the flavour and to make it look more attractive to eat. Some additives are "natural" substances, for example salt, some colourings, vitamin C, and lecithin. Additives are listed alongside ingredients on most packaged foods. Many additives are known by a European Union number—the "E" number. All the additives with E numbers have been tested for safety. The amount of an additive that is added to any one foodstuff is strictly controlled, but it is our own responsibility to notice amounts overall that we consume. A very small number of people are allergic to additives, but on the whole, you don't need to worry too much about them. The overall level that we take in from various sources, however, can be a reason for using fresh food when possible. Even fresh food needs careful washing before use, to keep down the amount of non-nutritional substances your body has to work at processing.

Managing a Healthy Weight

Underweight and overweight are states which are linked to food and physical activity. Food provides the energy—or calories—your body needs for all its processes, and for everyday physical activities such as breathing, sitting, standing and walking. If you don't eat enough food, or if you are not absorbing it properly, you may not be getting all the nutrients you need from your diet and you may become underweight. If the food you eat gives you more energy than you use, the extra is stored as fat, and you will put on weight. In Britain, more than 50% of the population is overweight and has too much body fat.

Your long-term condition may also be a factor in your weight.

It is not healthy to be either underweight or overweight. Deciding on what is a "healthy" weight for you is the task here! As a self-manager aiming at living a healthy life, this will be an area for review and action-planning, linked to, but not exactly the same as the review of your diet and your exercise programme. Again, brief notes on your calendar or in your journal will help you keep hold of the facts of the matter. Many of us do not have a rational or even a properly informed view of our weight. Now is a good time to tackle some of your own underlying issues based on the patterns you can see from your notes.

As usual, establishing a goal is a self-manager's first step, followed by listing options based on information gathered and acting on the plans made to try them out. By reviewing the success of the trials, you are well-placed to continue controlled changes. The rest of this chapter helps you to look at some of the common problems faced by many of us, to help you in your own action planning.

A healthy weight is the state in which you feel and function best physically and mentally, and in which you reduce your risk of developing or complicating health problems. Weight and fat aren't the same thing. Some of your weight is bone, muscle and so on; some of it is the water content of your body. Your weight varies according to your age and how much you move around, as well as how much you eat and drink. Probably you do not have one fixed healthy weight, too—you will be healthy and comfortable within a range of a few pounds. When you review your weight, consider these points and also take into account how much of your weight is fat, where the fat is on your body, and whether or not you have weight-related problems such as high blood pressure or a family history of such problems. Achieving and maintaining a healthy weight is important for everyone. As an aspect of symptom-management, weight can have a considerable impact on your disease. Excess fat around your waist is particularly risky. A waist circumference of more than 94cm (37 ins) in men and more than 80cm (32ins) in women has been associated with an increased risk of heart disease and diabetes.

The decision to change weight is a very personal one. To be told by someone else that you need to adjust your weight isn't the same as deciding yourself to take control. To help you decide whether or not you are ready to make any changes, think about some of the following points.

Taking Stock

For a rough guide, based on statistics from the general population, to whether you are a healthy weight, check your weight on the chart in Figure 12.2.

Making small, acceptable alterations to your diet and lifestyle can result in a gradual, sustained weight gain or loss—whichever is appropriate. For most people, any suggested weight adjustment programme will be in line with the Balance of Good Health. To maximise energy production through efficient absorption of nutrients, eat in a balanced way, as described in the first half of this chapter. People following a weight reducing diet may also be encouraged to watch the size of portions served, to eat regularly and not to skip meals. To make sure you are using up energy in physical activity, look back at the chapters on exercise and any notes you may have made in your journal. Walking more often, using the stairs instead of the lift, putting a bit more effort into housework and taking part in enjoyable activities such as golf or dancing are simple ways of being more active.

Use your consultants if you need more information or advice, beyond what your own information-gathering can tell you. Speak to your doctor, nurse or dietitian about what is a healthy weight for you, given your condition and treatment

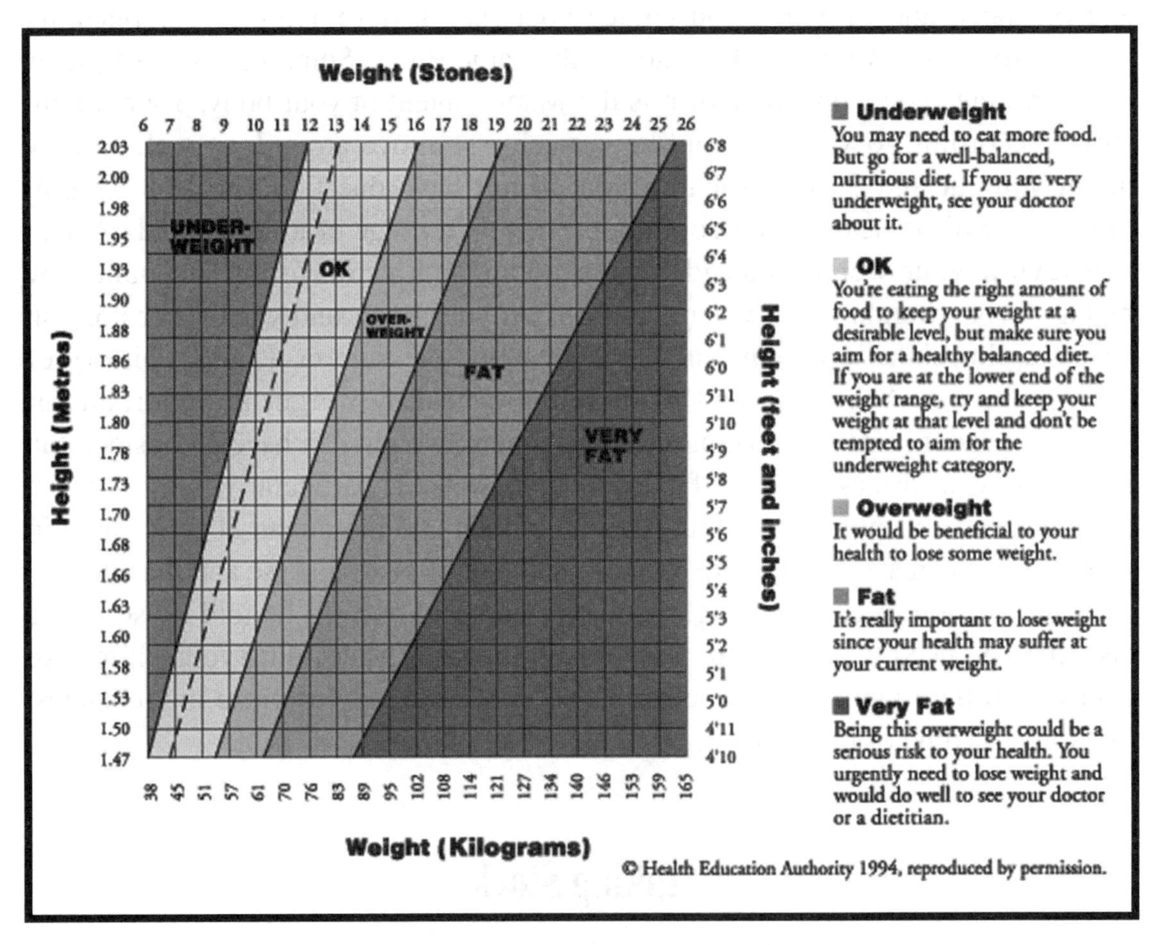

Figure 12.2 *Height/Weight Chart*

needs. You may already be at a healthy weight and need only to maintain it by eating well and staying active. If you would benefit from gaining or losing some weight, they will be able to help you in your action plans.

Why Change?

The reasons for losing or gaining weight are different for each individual. The most obvious reason may be your physical health, but there may also be psychological or emotional reasons for wanting to change. Consider why you want to change and record your answers, perhaps as shown below. You may find this helps when you come to review later whether you need to change your plans to solve a problem.

Write in your journal or on your calendar:

Changing my weight will help me . . .

- Lessen my disease symptoms
- Give me more energy to do the things I want to do
- Feel better about myself
- Change the way others perceive me
- Feel more in control of my disease and my life

or whatever else applies to you.

Change What?

If the two main ingredients for successful weight management are developing an active lifestyle and making changes in your eating patterns, consider carefully what each of these involves for you, from your work on the chapters on exercise, and the first part of this chapter. An active lifestyle implies doing some physical activity that burns calories and regulates appetite and metabolism, both important for weight management. Physical activity can also help you develop more strength and stamina, as well as move and breathe more easily. So you may find you need to change some things about your lifestyle. Activity doesn't wear you down or out, but actually boosts your energy level. Making changes in your eating habits may also be necessary. You would begin by making small, gradual changes in what you eat. This may mean changing the emphasis or quantity of certain foods you eat. This chapter should help.

Am I Ready?

Once you have reviewed your weight, and sorted out what needs doing, you are in a position to decide whether to make changes. If you consider your health would benefit by gaining or losing some weight, bear in mind the small changes suggested in the early part of this chapter. As we saw, you can implement some changes almost without noticing. If you combine consistent small changes with patience and perseverance, and assuming you do need to adjust your weight, there will be a change in your body eventually.

If, however, you decide that there is a large change to be made, such as we normally associate with "going on a diet", then it may be worth thinking through whether or not you are ready to do so. If you are not ready at this moment, you may be setting yourself up for failure. Success is important in weight management, because it is discouraging to go backwards. In the long run, it's not healthy eating or a balanced approach to let your weight "see-saw". So set things up for success by being sure you are ready to change.

Finish reading this chapter, which quotes some experiences around eating that you might recognise, and highlight in your self-management journal any of those which ring a bell with you. Change the phrasing if necessary to make it more exactly express your own experience. Add anything which is peculiar to your situation. There is no point in starting a project like a strict eating plan leaving unconsidered some major obstacle—work, money, family, a holiday—so this is the opportunity to consider it. There are suggestions in the chapter which you can reformulate into action plans to address the issues you identify.

If not now, fine—but when?

You may find that now is not the right time to start anything. If it is not, set a date in the future for a time when you will think again. In the meantime, accept that this is the right decision for you at this time, and focus your attention on other goals.

Starting Small—and Continuing Small

If you decide that now is the right time, start by changing those things that feel most comfortable to you. You don't have to do it all right away. Remember, slow and steady wins the race.

To help get started, keep track of what you are currently doing. For example, write down your daily routine to identify where you might be able to add some exercise. Or keep a food diary as part of your journal for a week to see what, when, why, and how much you eat. This can help you identify how and where to make changes in your eating habits, as well as how to shop for and prepare meals. The journal may also help you look at the relationship between your eating patterns and emotions or other symptoms. The sample food–mood diary on page 204 may be useful. Next, choose only one or two things to change first. Allow yourself time to get used to these and then add more changes. See if the goal setting and action planning skills discussed in Chapter 2 will help you with this.

Common Problems With Healthy Eating

"I enjoy eating out so how do I know if I'm eating well?"

If you don't have time, or you hate cooking, or you just don't have the energy to go grocery shopping and prepare meals, eating out may suit your needs.

Select restaurants that offer variety and flexibility in types of food and methods of preparation. Ask what's in a dish and how it's prepared, especially if you're eating in a restaurant where the dishes are new or different from what you're used to.

Plan what you will eat and how much. Look at the earlier part of the chapter for suggestions for eating balanced food when away from home. Choose dishes whose ingredients are listed. Instead of a whole dinner, order separate dishes and lots of vegetables—without butter or sauces. Watch portion sizes—maybe split a main meal or a dessert with someone else.

If you eat with others, order first so that you aren't tempted to change your order after hearing what they're having!

Choose salads with dressing on the side, baked potatoes instead of chips, juice or milk or water instead of soft and fizzy drinks.

"I snack while I watch TV or read."

If this is what you do, plan ahead by preparing healthier snacks—fresh fruit, raw vegetables, or popcorn without butter and sugar.

Try designating specific areas at home and work as "eating areas" and limit your eating to those areas.

"I eat when I'm bored." "I eat when I'm depressed." "I eat when I'm feeling lonely."

Many people find comfort in food. These are the times when celery sticks, apples, or popcorn don't seem to do the trick.

The feelings need exploring before the food habit can just fade away. Keep a food-mood diary for a week (page 204) or use your journal. Take this seriously

Food–Mood Diary

Date	Time	What I Ate	Where I Ate	Mood and Feelings

Things That Will Enable Me to Make the Desired Changes	**Things That Will Make It Difficult for Me to Change**
Example: I have the support of family and friends.	*Example:* The holidays are coming up and there are too many gatherings to prepare for.

and be honest with yourself. Every day, list what, how much, and when you eat. At the same time, try to work out what you are feeling when you have the urge to eat. If you can spot a pattern, write it down as a sentence and formulate a goal for an action plan. You may find you need to look at the way you are spacing your meals and snacks, too, as discussed in the first part of this chapter—a drop in your energy can lead to a feeling of depression. As you found in chapter 1, symptoms like these can be inter-related, so using your action plan is an effective way of breaking into the cycle of symptoms and linked behaviour.

Make an action plan for when these situations arise. Work out what you can do when you catch yourself feeling bored. Go for a short walk, work on a jigsaw puzzle, or otherwise occupy your mind and hands.

"Healthy food doesn't taste the same! The healthy stuff just doesn't fill me up!"

Eating in a balanced way will soon alter your perception of flavours. Sugar and salt can dominate your sense of taste, and when you reduce them, you can taste food properly. You free yourself to become aware of your hunger and your appetite in a different way, too. Non-nutritious food never satisfies, just because it is non-nutritious. Once your body is receiving the nutrition it needs, your hunger and your appetite become more trustworthy. (Really!)

Just because you are making healthier food choices does not mean that you will never again eat your favourite foods. You will find yourself happily eating in moderation.

"But I LOVE cooking!"

You're lucky. This is your opportunity to a cookery class or to buy a recipe book. Experiment with different ways with your favourite recipes, increasing the amount of fruit and vegetables you use and limiting the amount of fat, sugar and salt.

"I'm living alone now, and I'm not used to cooking for one. I find myself over-eating so food isn't wasted."

It might help to measure your ingredients for a week or two.

Don't put the serving dishes on the table. Take as much as you feel you can comfortably eat and bring only your plate to the table.

As soon as you've finished eating, wrap up what you haven't eaten and put it in the fridge or freezer. Then you have leftovers for the next day or whenever you don't want to cook.

Invite friends over for dinner once in a while so that you can share food and each other's company, or plan a potluck supper with neighbours or relatives.

Attend your community or church meals.

Common Problems With Losing Weight

"I wish I could lose ten pounds in the next two weeks. I want to look good for . . . ."

Sound familiar? People usually want to lose weight quickly. It may be possible to lose five to ten pounds (2–5 kg) in one or two weeks, but it's not healthy and it won't stay off. Rapid weight loss is usually water loss, which can be dangerously dehydrating. It can make you light-headed, tired, spoil your sleep and give you a headache. Use an orderly self-management approach. Use realistic goal-setting. Use positive self-talk.

Set your goal to lose weight gradually, just one or two pounds (1 kg) a week.

Identify the specific steps you will take to lose this weight, for example. You may increase your level of activity and do more, or you may make changes in what you eat, or both. Whatever they are, the changes will be considered, planned, recorded and reviewed.

Change your self-talk from "I really need to lose ten pounds right away" to "Losing this weight gradually will help me keep it off for good."

Be patient. You didn't gain weight overnight, so you can't expect to lose it overnight.

"The first several pounds go easily, but I can't seem to lose the last few."

This can be frustrating and puzzling, especially when you have been eating healthily and staying active. However, it is quite common and usually means that your body has adapted to your new calorie intake and activity level.

Take your action plan and move to the review step. Checking the results of your first option is step 5 of action planning. At this stage you look at what has happened so that you can identify what changes need making. While your first impulse may be to cut your calorie intake even further, it probably won't help and could be unhealthy. Ask yourself how much of a difference one, two, or even five pounds will really make. If you are feeling good, the chances are you don't need to lose more weight. You may already be at a healthy weight given your body size and shape. Also, you may be replacing fat with muscle, which weighs more.

Revise your goal. Perhaps aim to maintain your weight for a few weeks. Perhaps change the goal to a one pound a week weight loss, say. Work out your new action plan, so you know in detail what exactly you will do. When this is recorded, you will be in a position to re-review in a few weeks time on the basis of facts, not a panicky impulse.

Your action plan may include adding to your physical activity exercise goals, especially if what you are doing has become easy. Increasing your activity level will help you to use more calories and maintain your muscle mass. Less weight will be stored in the form of fat. Planning in detail will allow you to be patient and your body has time to adjust to your new patterns.

"I always feel so deprived of the foods I love when I try to lose weight."

Look at the foods you ARE going to eat. At the very least, list them, in detail. If it's possible, put a selection of them out on the table. There is more there than you could get through in weeks. When you have worked your way through trying them, trying new recipes, trying new combinations, then you may find you have a gap for some food you used to love—and you can have it.

The key to reaching and maintaining a healthy weight is to make changes you can tolerate, even enjoy. This means they must suit your lifestyle and needs.

"I eat too fast or I finish eating before everyone and find myself reaching for seconds."

- Maybe you are limiting yourself to only two or three meals a day, not eating or drinking between meals. This can leave you so hungry at mealtime that you practically inhale your food.
- Maybe you have not had a chance to slow down and relax before eating. Slowing yourself down slows your eating down, and that can help you decrease the amount of food you eat.
- Eat at every mealtime. You are less likely to overeat at the next meal.
- Eat a healthy snack between meals.
- Plan snacks for mid morning or afternoon. Fruit or raw vegetables carrot sticks make a good snack. These really do stave off the hunger pangs until your main meal.
- Eat more frequent, smaller meals.
- Chew your food well.
- Enjoy it.
- Drink water. You will feel better on six to eight glasses of water a day. Many people have to practise remembering to do this. Leave a glass poured where you will see it and keep count. Add this to what you normally drink. What happens is you begin to notice

thirst, quite possibly for the first time ever. A desire for a cup of tea is often a desire for water. Or you may want both. What's more, many people misinterpret the need for water as hunger. So although water doesn't stop you feeling hungry, you may find that it was water you needed all the time. On the whole, it's better not to drink a large amount at the same time as you eat. Half an hour before (or one minute before if your planning isn't that good) allows your body to absorb and use the water in the process of digestion.

- Try a relaxation method about half an hour before you eat. Several methods are discussed in chapter 5.

Common Problems With Gaining Weight

"I don't know how to add pounds."

There is far less information easily available in the media about gaining weight. The self-management task of gathering specific information may be demanding, and using your consultants may help at this stage. They might help you check that you are digesting food properly. In general, though, exactly the same principles apply. The Balance of Good Health balances both ways! There may be issues linked to your particular long-term condition so you could take this list of suggestions to your consultant to sort out exactly what is appropriate for you.

- Take as much care to tempt yourself with well-chosen, nicely-presented food as you would if you were looking after someone else.
- Keep to a routine so you don't forget to eat.
- Chew everything thoroughly.
- Increase the amount of calories and nutrients you eat. It may be appropriate to add fat in small regular quantities.
- Eat smaller meals more often during the day.
- Eat at all mealtimes.
- Eat high-calorie foods first at each meal, saving the vegetables and fruits till later.
- Don't drink at the same time as you eat.

- Use calorie-rich foods such as avocados, nuts, seeds, nut butter, or dried fruits for your snacks.
- Drink milk shakes, malt drinks, and fruit whips which are high in calories.
- Eat high-protein foods, such as meat, fish, nuts or dairy products.
- Use milk to prepare creamed dishes with meat, fish, or poultry.

- Add milk or milk powder to sauces, gravies, cereals, soups, and casseroles.
- Use melted cheese on vegetables and other dishes.
- Add butter, margarine, oils, and creams to dishes (1–3 tablespoons [15–45 ml] per day).
- Use protein, vitamin, and mineral supplements if needed. Get information from your consultant to find out what's best to use

"Food doesn't taste as good as before."

- Tackle any physical reason for your reduced enjoyment of the taste of food. Use your consultants to make sure your teeth, tongue, mouth and throat are as comfortable as possible.
- Aim to prepare your food to ease any physical problem you experience with eating. Juicers, liquidisers, blenders can improve the texture of many dishes without spoiling the flavours. Cutting small or grating can make many foods more accessible.
- Don't just add salt to improve the taste, because that will unbalance your intake of nutrients overall. Experiment with herbs, spices, and other seasonings, small amounts at a time A good handful of freshly chopped parsley on pasta is easy to do, delicious and much more interesting than salt.
- Chew your food well. This will allow the food to remain in your mouth longer and provide more stimulation to your taste buds.

"It takes so long to prepare meals. By the time I've done it, I'm too tired to eat."

If this is a problem for you, then it's time to develop a plan, because you need to eat to maintain your energy level. It is a priority because you are at risk of temptation otherwise, from a biscuit packet. Use action-planning to plan your meals for a week, buy the ingredients, and work out how you can divide your food preparation into steps during the day, resting in between.

Cook enough for two, three, or even more servings, especially if it's something you really like. Freeze the extra portions in single-serving sizes. On the days when you are really tired, thaw and reheat one of these pre-cooked, frozen meals.

Ask for help—make it a specific request. Do so especially for those big meals or at family gatherings.

"Sometimes eating causes discomfort." "I'm afraid I'll become short of breath while I'm eating."

People who experience shortness of breath or who find it difficult and physically uncomfortable to eat meals tend to eat less and may be underweight. Examine the exact reasons for your discomfort or your fear. Is the problem that you can't eat a large meal at one sitting? A full stomach reduces the space your breathing muscles have to expand and contract. This can aggravate breathing problems. Indigestible food sitting in the stomach for too long may also cause discomfort around breathing. Food which causes you to feel windy also puts pressure on your lungs.

Your action plan might work out in detail how to eat four to six smaller meals a day, rather than three larger meals. You reduce the amount of oxygen you need to chew and digest each meal.

- Avoid foods that produce wind or make you feel bloated. Record in your journal your experiments with different foods. The usual suspects tend to be vegetables such as cabbage, broccoli, brussels sprouts, some types of onion, beans and fruits like raw apples, melons, and avocados, especially if eaten in large quantities. Take them one at a time, give them a fair trial by chewing them thoroughly, and note which ones to avoid in future.
- Eat slowly. Eating quickly to avoid an episode of shortness of breath can actually bring one on. Slowing down and breathing evenly reduces the amount of air you swallow while eating.
- Take small mouthfuls.
- Chew your food well.
- Pause occasionally to breathe.
- Practise a relaxation exercise about half an hour before mealtime, or take time out for a few deep breaths during the meal.

"I can't eat much in one sitting."

- Eat four to six small meals in a day.
- Include "no fuss", high-calorie snacks like milk, bread, and fruits or liquid protein shakes.
- Eat the portion of your meal that is highest in calories first. Save the vegetables and fruits till the end—but do eat them!

Common Problems With Maintaining Weight

"I've been on a LOT of diets before and lost a lot of weight. But it's always come back, with extra on top. It's so frustrating, and I don't understand WHY this happens!!!"

Many of us have shared this experience. Diets which proceed like this are not balanced, and that's why they fail. When we undertake them, we are not balanced, either. Or at least, there is a sort of balance, because in this case what goes down must come up! Nothing has changed permanently, and as we go back to eating in our old way, so the weight must come back too.

Very likely the diets were short-term and their approach was to restrict calories. They would not have emphasised steady, long-term changes in eating habits. The change would only have been intended for a limited period. They probably demanded sudden, drastic changes in both what you ate and the way you ate it.

You can't tolerate a diet like this for long. Because your body does not know when food will be available again, it reacts physiologically to being deprived. It slows your metabolism to adapt to a smaller amount of energy from the reduced amount of food. Your weight loss slows, too. Then, at some low point, the swing back will have begun. Either your body decides that you must eat more and you find yourself stuffing food down your throat, or you reach your arbitrary target weight. Back you go to your old way of eating. Back comes the weight. The scales literally tip the other way.

Possibly you put on even more weight than you lost. It seems likely that the body responds self-defensively in this situation. It replenishes its stores, usually in the form of fat, to be called on again for energy next time the calories are restricted. The presence of this fat causes a further unbalanced response when you decide consciously that you really have to get on top of this. You begin yet another sudden, and, to your subconscious mind, dangerous restriction on food. So the weight goes down and up in cycles which are unhealthy and extremely discouraging. You were probably aware of a sense of deprivation. You couldn't have what you wanted. But you very likely didn't realise how profound that feeling is. It's a survival issue. So now after the stringent diet has slipped, we eat everything we think we want, defiantly and more of it—and the balance of the weight goes right over the top again.

The recommendations in this chapter are focused on balancing—weighing up problems, weighing up solutions, observing and recording effects, balancing nutrients, balancing food groups, and giving proper attention to the feelings which underlie unbalanced eating. Your aim is change slowly and gradually, using your mind to manage the process, allowing time for the body to adjust—whether you are gaining weight, losing it, or on a comfortable lifetime maintenance programme firmly based on good food. You do not need to swing one way or the other any more. You can be in control of your food, and how it is prepared and served, and "yo-yo" dieting is a thing of the past.

Keep an eye on your activity level. Once you have lost some weight, exercise three to five times a week improves your chances of keeping the weight off. Even, if possible, do a bit more.

"I do all right maintaining my weight for a short time. Then something happens beyond my control, and my concerns about what I eat become insignificant. Before I know it I've slipped back into my old eating habits."

If there was just a little slip, don't worry about it. Carry on with your original successful maintenance programme as if nothing happened.

If it's more than a slip, you might choose to view it as a "problem" and sit down to do some fresh action planning. Has some event or situation arisen which has taken your mind off your food choices? If so, weight management may have taken a back seat for a while. Whatever's going on round you, which may feel out of your control, needs accommodating by you and that takes energy and attention. You might interpret this interruption as a set-back, but it need not appear so and may not be so. Every change we make sets more change in action, often moving us forward.

Using an action-planning procedure, however, is within our control, and sitting down and contemplating our current situation is possible and helpful. You may find you can return to your diet or you may identify new goals and new options to move things on.

One option might be to increase your network of consultants by looking for a local diet support group. Check their credentials for balance, though! Make sure they emphasise good nutrition from a wide variety of foods and that they emphasise changes in eating habits and patterns. If the group's advice relies on your eating some special meal or supplement, don't join. You would want proper support in the form of meetings or long-term follow-up.

Eating healthily does not mean cutting out things you like. It means learning to eat a variety of foods in the right quantities and at the right times to maintain your health and better manage your disease symptoms. The Balance of Good Health emphasises eating a wide variety of foods in moderation. When you choose to modify your diet to lose weight, to gain weight or to maintain weight, you are not punishing yourself. As a self-manager, you are freely making changes to find what is best for you. And if you really want to, you can do it!

• • •

Suggested Further Reading

British Heart Foundation. *The Light-Hearted Cookbook and The Everyday Light-Hearted Cookbook*. London: British Heart Foundation. Write to BHF, 14 Fitzharding Street, London W1H 6DH. Tel: 010 7935 0185

British Heart Foundation. "So you want to lose weight . . . for good." British Heart Foundation, 14 Fitzardinge Street, LondonW1H 6DH. Tel 0207 935 0185.

Escott-Stump, Sylvia. *Nutrition and Diagnosis-Related Care*. Lippincott Williams and Wilkins, 1997.

Hodgkin, John E. (Editor), et al. *Pulmonary Rehabilitation*. Lippincott Williams and Wilkins.

Peters, James A., Kenneth Burke, and Debra White. "Nutrition and the pulmonary patient." In *Pulmonary Rehabilitation: Guidelines to Success*, edited by John E. Hodgkin, Eileen G. Zorn, and Gerilynn L. Conners. Stoneham, Mass.: Butterworth Publishers, 1984

Other Resources

There is so much information available commercially and on the Internet on diets and healthy eating that it is sometimes difficult to know what to believe. The website, www.quackwatch.com is useful to check claims made about food supplements. Other resources include:

The Food Standards Agency has various leaflets on food related issues. See http://www.foodstandards.gov.uk

NHS Direct online www.nhsdirect.nhs.uk has a great deal of information on healthy eating, diet and nutrition

The press generally keeps a watchful eye on diet and health issues. The BBC website is a good way to keep up with health in the news, www.bbc.co.uk/health/nutrition

Most GP surgeries and health centres have information on general diets and special diets for people with certain conditions

CHAPTER 13

Managing Your Medicines

When you have a chronic illness, you are quite likely to be taking one or more medicines for a long time. As an active self-manager, it's important to understand what you're taking and why, so that you manage that area of your life efficiently.

If you are thinking "But my doctor decides my medicines," then you are alert to an apparent contradiction. How can you manage your medicines if your doctor is the expert?

The answer is that when you see your doctor, you are working in partnership. You have your job, they have theirs. Neither can operate without active and thoughtful co-operation from the other. What this chapter is intended to do is to outline your role and give you the opportunity to review your circumstances, your knowledge and information, and your goals, in relation to managing your medicines.

Medicines—What Do You Think?

We have a complicated relationship with medicines. It is only recently that the term "medicine" has been reserved for chemicals taken as a therapy, and the term "drug" reserved for chemicals taken without medical supervision or illegally. What we are prescribed by the doctor is a "medicine". The "drug" or "pharmaceutical" companies inform doctors and supply pharmacies and hospitals. They supply us with "over-the-counter" drugs which we can buy. Some of these have to be paid for by some people, some are free. Some drugs which used to be prescribed can now be bought freely from a chemist or a pharmacy or even a supermarket. For some of these—paracetamol for example—there is no age limit on the purchaser, though other drugs—alcohol and nicotine—can't be bought by young people. What's more these are seldom referred to as drugs. Herbal medicines, using a whole plant from which a prescribed drug may be extracted, are for sale in shops, or practitioners of herbal medicine can prescribe them. Cannabis, a plant like many other herbal medicines, though alleged to have curative properties, can't be bought legally anywhere and is known as an illegal drug. Drugs related to cocaine and heroin, which are illegal substances if they change hands for private "recreational" use, are used legally in hospitals to relieve suffering. Caffeine is freely available and legal, an inextricable part of our whole social fabric. "Under the influence of drugs" or "on drugs" suggests a level of irresponsibility, and even illegality, although anyone taking a medicine is arguably under the influence of drugs and yet is doing nothing illegal. Medicines for sale "over-the-counter"—OTC—are advertised and promoted. Ibuprofen, for instance, is marketed in a number of different smart packages with claims that it relieves pain. Some prescription-only medicines may not be advertised but many—Viagra for impotence and statins for cardiovascular disease—hit the headlines and appear in news items and magazine feature articles. The public is given a lot of partial and incomplete information and we often don't sit and consider exactly what we think. Steering a path through all this is not easy.

A good guide is your pharmacist. Be aware of the resource available to you in your local chemist or pharmacy. Pharmacists are highly-trained professionals. They know how drugs work in the body and are familiar with possible drug interactions—that is, the effects two drugs may cause when they're in your system at the same time. Pharmacists frequently advise doctors and can also advise you. You should find it easy to talk to your local pharmacist—they are usually ready to discuss your medicine with you. Sometimes the conversation may be a bit public, but if you find it awkward, just ask for a quiet word about whatever your question is. Many pharmacists value direct contact with patients and are a mine of information. Pharmacists—dispensing chemists as they used to be called—increasingly serve the public in this way. It's a good idea to find a pharmacist you like and to stay with them. Gradually they will build up a picture of your medicine requirements and be in a good position to advise you when asked. As a self-manager, don't forget the pharmacists. They are helpful consultants.

One of our jobs as self-managers is to explore our own attitude to the medicine we take. Underlying our desire for, or aversion to, medicine are some complex feelings, based on experience and knowledge, or lack of them! Our perception of what our medicine does, and whether it works at all, is often subjective, and it can be coloured by these hidden feelings. Work out where you stand yourself as a first step to managing your medicines. As with other self-management areas of our lives, this one will benefit from periodic review, and possibly for change, to make sure you are always managing things to your benefit. You might also look at the section later in this chapter about remembering to take your medicines—it suggests some questions to ask yourself which are relevant here.

Although we tend to think of taking medicine to make us better, medicines don't actually cure us. In the most practical way, your body is its own healer. Even if you take medicine, it's still only helping the body. Given time, some symptoms and disorders improve, and one treatment option for you and your doctor is simply to wait and watch. Patience, careful self-observation and monitoring can be very therapeutic.

Effects of Medicines—What They Do

But it is also true that medicines can be a very important part of the management of a chronic illness. Although medicines do not cure a disease they can help people live with it, by doing various jobs.

- Through their chemical action in the body, they act to counter symptoms. Medicine delivered via a bronchodilator inhaler expands the airways and make it easier to breathe.
- Another function is to prevent further problems. Medicines that thin the blood help prevent blood clots and reduce risk of a second stroke.
- A third job is to improve symptoms or to slow the disease process. Non-steroidal anti-inflammatory medicines—NSAIDs—can help arthritis by quieting the inflammatory process.
- Some medicines are replacements for substances that the body is no longer producing adequately. Insulin is provided as a medicine for someone with diabetes.
- In all cases, the purpose of a medicine is to make your life in some way more manageable.

So, any medicine you are taking will be doing one or more of these jobs. As you read in chapter 4, *Understanding and Managing Common Symptoms*, the symptoms suffered by one person may be complicated. They are often inter-related. One very good reason for knowing which medicine you are taking and why, is to help you sort out the tangle and perhaps break the cycle of symptom causes and effects. In the relationship with your doctor, you are the partner with responsibility for feeding back accurately. If you have understood what the medicine was intended to do, the more precisely you can tell your doctor about its action and the better their next prescription can be.

Keeping Track of Effects

It would be an ideal world where causes and effects were simple and visible and the reality is that it's hard to be sure what does what. A medicine is only one part of the complicated pattern of your life. But this needn't stop you trying to sort out the strands. A log of your procedures and progress on a calendar, or the journal about your symptoms and your diet may be, again, a valuable resource for you and your doctor. If you know exactly what you began taking on which day, you can both have a better notion of whether an improvement was linked to that medicine or not.

It may be the case, for example, that you think a medicine is doing nothing. The temptation might be to stop taking it. If you have understood from the start that this medicine's job is to slow the course of your disease, you will be far better placed to trust your doctor and carry on as agreed. It can be important to continue taking your medicines, even if you have no direct evidence of how they are helping. Equally, you will be better placed to ask for a review of the prescription if you know exactly how long you have taken it, and to understand what the doctor says at this point.

Placebo Effect—Body and Mind

Trusting your doctor, from a strong position of good communication and good information, can be a very important part of the management of your condition, and of the healing process. Trusting your medicine matters, as well.

This does not mean that you unquestioningly swallow anything you are given, either literally or metaphorically. Quite the opposite, in fact. Asking your questions, gathering your information, being an active participant in your healing process from the start allows you to be sure that the medicine you take is the best in the circumstances, and that you can expect the best from it.

Your expectation about what the medicine can do for you is more important than we once thought. Traditionally, we took a pill to stop a symptom. We would have expected to be able to say, "Yes, it's worked" or "No, it's done nothing".

However, a great deal of research has shown that what we expect of a treatment actually influences its outcome. Your beliefs and expectations for the medicine can change your body chemistry and so affect how the medicine works on your symptoms. This input from your mind results in what is called the "placebo effect."

Thousands of scientific studies have shown that people suffering from a wide variety of diagnosed ailments have improved after taking a plain unmedicated pill, believing it to be an active drug. About one-third of patients in such studies reported improvements. Placebos have relieved headaches, ulcers, asthma, arthritis, hay fever, colds, warts, constipation, angina, insomnia, and pain after surgery—all undeniably physical ailments. Cholesterol levels, blood pressure, blood counts, gastric acidity, and overall immune function have been altered by taking a placebo.

People used to discount this effect as evidence of people's suggestibility, but looked at the other way, suggestibility can be used to your advantage. The proof of the power of mind is deeply significant. It is very important indeed to someone with a chronic condition to know that there is scientific evidence of the immense power of belief. Chapter 5 suggests deliberately accessing and, through regular practice, developing the power of your mind. Belief isn't something that lucky people are born with—it's a conscious decision to act in a certain way. This is exactly what people who decide to manage their lives with a long-term condition have done. Using your mind as a powerful resource can improve many aspects of your situation, and the medicines your doctor offers you are no exception. Taking a medicine you have informed yourself about, in partnership with a doctor you trust, can enhance your self-healing mechanisms in more ways than just biochemical.

It is as if our positive beliefs and expectations switch on our self-healing mechanisms. When you review your feelings about medicine, examine the beliefs you have about your treatment. If you tell yourself, "I'm not a pill taker," or, "Medicines always give me bad side effects," your body is likely to follow the lead of your mind. Instead you can use the power of your mind to counteract habitual negative images by replacing them in visualisations with vital, lively and health-promoting ones. Perhaps you find it easier to associate healthy images with vitamins than with medicines. Each vitamin pill affirms that you are doing something positive to prevent disease and promote health. Extend this image to the medicines you choose to take as well. You can also choose to use positive self-talk. This can transform your "normal" frame of mind. Have a look at chapter 5

Imagine how the medicine is helping you. Develop a mental image of how it is helping your body. Perhaps a thyroid hormone replacement can be visualised filling a missing link in your body's chemical chains, balancing and regulating your metabolism. An antibiotic might be seen as a strong broom sweeping germs out of the body. Don't worry if your image of what's happening is not 100% physiologically correct. It's the effect of a clear, positive image that counts. Positive self-talk backs this up. "I am supporting my immune system with this pill." "This pill is keeping the swelling down so I have more energy to keep moving and get strong." Keep in mind why you are taking the medication. "Because my doctor told me to" is not nearly as effective as understanding how the medication can help you and deciding to use it positively. "Because I have decided to" is a much stronger starting point, and "Because I know it will help me" can be a self-fulfilling prophecy.

Knowing that the way the medicine works 'fits' with your ideas about what needs to happen inside your body to manage the disease or the symptoms seems to be the basis for the placebo effect. Ask your doctor or pharmacist 'what does this medicine do?' If their explanation doesn't make sense, or doesn't fit with your ideas, tell them.

Side-Effects

Nearly all medicines have some effects beyond the one you want, and those you don't want are called side-effects. Medicines can be immensely effective, but we pay a price for having such powerful tools. Some side-effects are predictable and minor, a few are unexpected and life-threatening. From 5% to 10% of all hospital admissions are due to side-effects of medicines or to medicine reactions. So if you are taking one or more medicines, you need to know about the medicine's intended effect and its possible side-effects, to avoid making mistakes in how you take it, and to be better prepared to tell your doctor about your progress.

Sometimes people say, quite reasonably, they can't or won't take a medicine because of possible side-effects, but such a decision needs to be based on information from your doctor, your pharmacist and the patient information leaflet that comes with the medicine. You may decide that the benefits from a medicine outweigh the side-effects. The use of chemotherapy for people with cancer is a good example. The medicines undoubtedly have side-effects, but many people still choose to take them because they can save lives. To take or not to take a medicine is your decision, but approach the decision positively by asking yourself, "Will I be better off with the medicine despite its side effects?"

There could be ways of avoiding the side-effects or making them less severe. The way you take the medicine can make a difference. Ask your doctor or pharmacist for advice on this question, and consider what they say in relation to your own situation.

There is likely to be an alternative medicine with the same benefits and fewer side-effects. Your doctor may be able to try several medicines to find one that is best for you. Try out a prescription for a week or two before moving to a month's supply so that you don't waste time and money.

Taking several medicines at the same time could complicate side-effects. Patients with multiple problems will often be prescribed multiple medicines. You may be taking something to lower your blood pressure, an anti-inflammatory for arthritis, a pill for angina, a bronchodilator for asthma, antacids for heartburn, a tranquilliser for anxiety, plus a handful of over-the-counter remedies and herbs. The more medicines you are taking, the greater the risk of side effects. As you get to grips with managing your medication, you can probably be more exact about what needs treating and so cut down the number of medicines and the associated risks. You need a good partnership with your doctor and maybe your pharmacist, so that you can actively take part in decisions about what to take and for how long.

Getting the Best from Your Medicine

Your response to a particular medicine depends on your age, metabolism, activity level, the other medicines you're taking, and the pattern of your symptoms. You need to work out a plan for yourself with your doctor or your pharmacist. Many medicines are prescribed on a "PRN" basis—PRN is short for the Latin words meaning "when necessary". That means that you are the one who decides what's necessary, so you judge when to take it, how much you need and when to stop. Your doctor relies on you to report effects and side effects. Depending on what you say, your doctor may change the medicine or the dose, or stop it altogether.

You can see how the partnership between you and your doctor needs to work. You tell them things and find things out from them. Sometimes, unfortunately, it doesn't work like this. Very very few patients actually ask questions to find out about new prescriptions. Doctors tend to think, understandably, that silence means you are clear about everything and happy. When things do go wrong, it can often be tracked back to patients not knowing enough about the medicine itself. They may also not have understood how to take the medicine. You really do have to know what you're taking, for the medicine to be as safe and as effective as possible, so you need to ask questions until you're sure you've understood. People don't like asking questions, in case they look ignorant or challenging. But asking questions clearly and politely, and listening carefully to the answers, is a necessary part of a healthy doctor–patient relationship and it's certainly essential to successful and responsible self-management. Your confidence as a questioner will grow with practice!

The goal of treatment is to maximise the benefit and minimise the risks. This means taking the fewest medicines, in the lowest effective doses, for the shortest period of time. Don't sit back and let the doctor do it—do everything you can to help yourself.

Tell Your Doctor

Even if your doctor doesn't ask, there are things you should tell them.

- **Are you taking any medicines?** Take along to your doctor a complete list of all your pills, tablets, liquid medicine, capsules, powders, inhalers, everything. That means copying down the actual name of the medicine from the box, and the dose. Tell them the whole lot, including birth control pills, vitamins, aspirin, antacids, laxatives, herbal remedies and things you have bought for yourself. If you've seen a doctor in a hospital and they have prescribed, don't forget that. This really matters if you are seeing more than one prescriber otherwise they won't know what the other has given you. If you're complaining of dizziness, say, the doctor needs to know which medicines you are taking, in case together they are known to cause dizziness. The doctor will treat that differently from dizziness that comes from an ear problem. There may be occasional prescribers too—if you see a dentist and they give you antibiotics, mention that, and tell the dentist what you are taking as well. If you write a list of all the medicines you are taking and their dosages, it can save your doctor time. Your pharmacist would find it useful as well.
- **Have you had allergic or unusual reactions to any medicines?** Describe any symptoms or unusual reactions you have had to any medicines taken in the past. Say exactly which medicine and what type of reaction. A rash, high temperature or wheezing that develops after taking a medicine is often an allergic reaction. The severity of allergic reactions can vary considerably. If any of these occur, call your doctor at once. But nausea, ringing in the ears, light-headedness and agitation are more likely to be side effects rather than an allergic reaction. Again, speak to your doctor.

- **Do you have any major chronic diseases or other medical conditions?** Tell your doctor what your condition is, even if it seems completely obvious to you, especially the first couple of times you see them. They need to know what you are suffering from, before they can prescribe. If there's something wrong with your liver or kidneys, mention this, because they are involved in the absorption, distribution and detoxification of the medicines you take. Your doctor may avoid certain medicines if you've got, or have had, hypertension, peptic ulcer, asthma, heart disease, diabetes, or prostate problems. Also say if you might be, or are, pregnant and if you're breast-feeding since many medicines aren't safe for use then.

- **What medicines were tried in the past to treat your disease?** Keeping a record of what you have taken in the past, and what your reactions were, can help your doctor choose a medicine now. The calendar log or journal suggested several times earlier in this book could be valuable now, too. One point—just because a medicine didn't do what you wanted in the past does not mean it can't be tried again. Diseases change and may become more responsive to treatment.

Ask Your Doctor

- **Do I really need this medicine?** Sometimes doctors prescribe because they think this is what patients expect. They feel pressure to do something for the patient because they want to help. Don't pressurise your doctor for medicines. The ones you may have heard about are likely to be new and in the newspapers, but some new drugs are promoted by pharmaceutical companies before the full range of hazards is known—they have even, occasionally, been withdrawn from use. You can choose to consider it good news if your doctor doesn't prescribe a medicine. It is much more likely to be that than a sign of rejection or lack of interest. Sometimes the best medicine is none at all and a decision by you and your doctor to wait and watch can be the wisest course.

  As you develop your action plans, your may find for yourself that lifestyle changes such as exercise, diet and stress management can, and will be your choice. When any treatment is recommended, ask what the likely consequences are if you postpone treatment so that you can decide to try a lifestyle change for a while. Many conditions can be treated in a variety of ways, and your doctor can explain alternative choices—perhaps ask about herbs and other non-medicine alternatives.

- **What is the name of the medicine?** If a medicine is prescribed, learn its name. Write down both the brand name and the generic or chemical name and memorise how to say it. If the medicine you get from the pharmacy doesn't have the same name as the one your doctor prescribed, ask the pharmacist to explain the difference.
- **What is the medicine supposed to do?** Your doctor should tell you why the medicine is being prescribed and how it might be expected to help you. It may be intended to prolong your life, completely or partially relieve your symptoms, or improve your ability to function. For example, if you are given a diuretic for high blood pressure, the medicine is probably intended to prevent later complications, rather than to stop your headache. On the other hand, if you are given paracetamol, the purpose is to help ease pain. Your doctor will tell you also how soon you can expect results from the medicine. Some medicines which treat infections or inflammation may take several days to a week to show improvement, while antidepressant medicines and some arthritis medicines typically take several weeks to begin working. On the other hand some medicines start to have a noticeable effect immediately.
- **How and when do I take the medicine and for how long?** You need to know how much and how often to take it for the medicine to be safe and effective. If the instruction says, "every six hours", sort out whether it means "every six hours while awake" or "every six hours and set an alarm to take some in the night as well." Should the medicine be taken before meals, with meals, or between meals? What should you do if you accidentally miss a dose? Should you skip it, take a double dose next time, or take it as soon as you remember? Should you continue taking the medicine until the symptoms subside or until the medicine is finished?

The answers to such questions are important. For example, if you are taking a non-steroidal anti-inflammatory medicine for arthritis, you may feel better within a few days, but should still take the medicine as prescribed to maintain the anti-inflammatory effect. Or, if you abruptly stop taking steroid medicines used for severe asthma as soon as the wheezing improves, you are likely to relapse. If you are using an inhaled medicine for treatment of asthma, the way you use the inhaler determines how much of the medicine actually gets into your lungs. Taking the medicine properly is vital, but patients don't always feel that they have been told clearly what to do. If you feel like that, ask your doctor or your pharmacist. They won't mind explaining it again. And again, if necessary!

- **What foods, drinks, other medicines, or activities should I avoid while taking this medicine?** The presence of food in the stomach may help protect the stomach from some medicines while it may render other medicines ineffective. For example, milk products or antacids block the absorption of the antibiotic tetracycline, so this medicine is best taken on an empty stomach. Some medicines may make you more sensitive to the sun, putting you at increased risk of sunburn. Ask whether the medicine prescribed will interfere with driving safely. Other medicines you may be taking, even over-the-counter medicines and alcohol, can either amplify or inhibit the effects of the prescribed medicine. Taking aspirin along with an anti-coagulant medicine can result in enhanced blood-thinning and possible bleeding. The more medicines you are taking, the greater the chance of an undesirable medicine interaction. So talk to your pharmacist about possible medicine-medicine and medicine-food interactions.

- **What are the most common side-effects, and what should I do if they occur?** All medicines have side-effects. You need to know what symptoms to be on the lookout for and what action to take if they develop. Ought to you to treat it as an emergency, discontinue the medicine, keep taking the medicine or call your doctor? While your doctor can't be expected to tell you every possible adverse reaction, they should talk to you about the more common and important ones. Ask specifically about precautions you should take, and the possible side-effects of any new medicine you are prescribed. If your doctor doesn't volunteer the information, it is up to you to raise the question.

- **Do I need tests to monitor the effects of this medicine?** You and your doctor mostly monitor the effect of a medicine personally by discussing if you're better or not, and that generally means discussing what your symptoms tell you. However, some medicines can disrupt body chemistry before any telltale symptoms develop. You might need a laboratory test, like a blood count or a liver function test, to alert you in advance of symptoms. You might also need a test to measure the amount of medicine in your blood, to arrive at a correct dose for you. Ask your doctor if the medicine being prescribed will need follow-up tests like these.

- **Could I have an alternative or generic medicine that is less expensive?** Every medicine has at least two names, a generic name and a brand name. The generic name is the name used to refer to the medicine in the scientific literature. The brand name is the company's unique name for the medicine. When a pharmaceutical company develops a new medicine, they are granted exclusive rights to produce it for seventeen years. In this time they will recover the costs of developing it. After seventeen years, other companies may market chemical equivalents of that medicine. These generic medicines are considered as safe and effective as the original brand-name, but often cost half as much. Doctors in general practice and in hospitals are encouraged to use generics to keep medicine costs down. Sometimes it is cheaper for you to buy the appropriate OTC medicine over-the-counter rather than paying the prescription charge. The medicine is just as good. The guidance on how and when to take it should be followed as closely as before.

- **Who else can I ask about the medicine?** Realistically, your doctor may not have time to go into all your questions in great detail and anyway it's difficult for anyone to remember all the answers. All medicines come with a patient information leaflet. Some of these are excellent and will give you an advice line to call for further information. Some leaflets are very legalistic and list every side effect that has ever happened to anyone, anywhere. So read them carefully but don't imagine it's all going to happen to you. Consult your pharmacist, who'll probably be able to tell you more. There are also useful websites, for example www.femail.co.uk and www.medicine-chest.co.uk that you can go to for information.

Even when you know a lot about a medicine it's worth getting the pharmacist's opinion. Sometimes specialist nurses are available by phone for advice about your medicines or phone voluntary organisations' helplines—they usually have leaflets. There are many sources of information and advice available. Some useful books are listed at the end of the chapter.

Prescriptions and Prescription Charges (As of June 2007)

NHS prescriptions cost £6.85 per item and are dispensed by the community pharmacist. That can add up. You may be able to keep the costs down.

Check that you have to pay at all. There are several exemptions. You are automatically exempt if you are:

- Under 16
- Under 19 and in fulltime education
- 60 or over
- Getting income support or income based Job Seekers Allowance
- Getting a maximum award of working families tax credit, or a disabled person's tax credit or the amount taken off the maximum is £71 per week or less
- The partner (or dependent child) of someone who gets one of the benefits in the above list
- You are an asylum seeker getting government support, or their partner or dependent child

You also qualify for an exemption certificate if you are:

- An expectant mother
- A woman who had a child in the last year
- Someone with a specified condition or are housebound with a continuing disability
- A war service pensioner needing treatment of accepted disabilities

- Or qualify under the low income scheme

Specified conditions are:

- A permanent physical disability that prevents you from leaving your home except with the help of someone else
- Fistulas or stomas that require dressings or an appliance
- Diabetes when the control is not by diet alone
- Conditions where supplemental thyroid hormone is necessary
- Epilepsy requiring continuous anti-convulsive therapy
- Hyperthyroidism, hypopituitism, myasthenia gravis and hypoadrenalism

The forms needed to claim these exemptions come from the pharmacist. The pharmacist is required to ask you for evidence that you qualify for an exemption.

Another way of reducing your prescription charges is to buy a prepayment certificate. These cover all your prescription costs for the relevant period. A four month prepayment certificates costs £31.90 and a year certificate costs £87.60. These certificates save you money if you need more than fourteen items a year or more than five prescriptions in four months. There is just one snag. There is a ceiling on the income you can have and be entitled to these certificates. However the calculation is complex and does not apply to most people.

Don't try to claim exemption from prescription charges if you aren't entitled to it. Prescription forms are audited and false declarations are followed up. However, make sure that you do claim all you can. Read the exemptions on the form carefully. If you have questions about your entitlement, ask the pharmacist. You can get quite a lot of help from the state if you spend time and thought on working out your benefits entitlement. Read the small print, ask in the pharmacy, get a calculator and do the sums properly, and you may find you can be financially better off than you thought.

Remembering to Take Your Medicine

No medicine will do you any good if you don't take it. Nearly half of all medicines are not taken regularly as prescribed. People forget, don't have clear instructions, find the dosing too complicated, don't like the side-effects, don't like or can't afford prescription charges, believe it won't do any good. And so on. Whatever the reason, if you have trouble taking your medicines as prescribed, talk to your doctor. Often, simplifying the process can make it easier. You might be able to come off one medicine, or take doses at different times. You may also find that reviewing your whole medicine pattern and looking at the feelings and beliefs you have, as discussed earlier in this chapter, can reveal underlying problems that need solving differently.

And, as an active self-manager, you have already realised that understanding more about your medicines can motivate you to take them regularly.

I forgot to take it—again. Why?

Ask yourself the following questions, and look at the answers for the review stage of your action plan. You'll need to talk to your doctor about much of this although the first few questions may allow you confront, and transform, some of your underlying beliefs yourself.

- Are you embarrassed about taking the medicine?
- Do you view taking the medicine as a sign of weakness or failure?
- Do think people might judge you negatively if they knew about it?
- Do you understand the instructions for how and when to take the medicine?
- Do you find the timetable for taking your medications too complicated?
- Are you disturbed by side effects?
- Is your medicine too expensive?
- Do you feel your disease is not serious enough to need regular medicine?
- Do you feel that the treatment is unlikely to help?
- Have you had a bad experience with medicine, either this one or another before now?
- Do you know someone else who had a bad experience with the medicine?
- Are you afraid of becoming addicted to the medicine?

- Do you tend to be forgetful anyway?

List some options for an action plan to remind you. There are some suggestions in chapter 16, *Helpful Hints*, gathered from many people who have found ways round exactly the practical problems you may face.

Practical Medicine Management

Over the counter medicines

You are your own medicine manager. Sometimes you will buy medicine for yourself, over the counter (OTC). For an OTC medicine, you should know, just as with medicine from your doctor, what you are taking, why, and how to use it wisely.

- Read OTC medicine labels and patient information leaflets and follow directions carefully. The label must by law include names and quantities of the active ingredients, safety precautions, and directions for use.
- Check with the pharmacist before buying it—it's a situation where a list of your medicines, as suggested above, might be useful. These medicines have a chemical effect on your body, just the same as prescribed medicines, and can react with other drugs in your system at the time. You can cancel out another medicine, or you can exaggerate the effect of, say, alcohol, by mixing what you take. Don't take more than it says, and leave the proper time between doses. If possible, select medicines with single active ingredients rather than combination "all-in-one" products so as not to risk side-effects of medicines you may not even need. Single-ingredient products also allow you to adjust the dosage of each medicine so you get maximum benefit with least risk of side-effects.
- Never take or give a medicine from an unlabelled container or a container whose label you can't read. Keep your medicines in their original labelled containers or transfer them to a labelled medicine organiser or pill dispenser. Don't make the mistake of mixing different medicines in the same bottle "just for now".

- Do not take medicines left over from a previous illness or that were prescribed for someone else, even if you have similar symptoms. Don't give your medicine to anyone else. Always check with your doctor or pharmacist that your medicine is the right one for you now.

- Pills can sometimes get stuck in the oesophagus, the "feeding tube" from your mouth down your throat. Sometimes your pill goes down more easily with well-chewed food, or drink at least a half glass of water with your pills and remain standing or sitting upright for a few minutes after swallowing. Some medicines are best taken on an empty stomach, and some fruit juices interact with some medicines. Check with your pharmacist the best way to swallow your specific tablets or capsules.

- If you are pregnant or breast-feeding, if you have a chronic condition, or are already taking multiple medicines, ask your pharmacist or your doctor to check that the OTC medicine you've chosen is safe.

- Store your medicines in a safe place away from the reach of any children. Children are curious and can get to places you don't expect. Poisoning with medicines is a distressingly common problem and completely preventable. Use a locked box—a small tool chest or a fishing box might suit you.

- The bathroom is not a particularly good place to store medicines. It can be relatively public. The atmosphere is often steamy and medicines need to be kept dry.

- Many medicines have an expiry date of two or three years. Get rid of all expired, past their use-by medicines by taking them to the pharmacy for safe disposal. Do not flush them away because unnecessary chemicals are best kept out of the water systems.

See chapter 16 *Helpful Hints* for some practical tips.

Medicines can help you or harm you. By exercising your skills as an active self-manager you can use medicines helpfully to make your life easier. Knowing your medicines and knowing your doctor, can allow medicines to act the best way they can.

• • •

Suggested Further Reading

Blair, Pat. *Know Your Medicines*. London: Age Concern Books, 1997.

Henry, John A. *BMA Medicines and Drugs*, 5th ed. London: Dorling Kindersley, 2000.

Henry, John A. *The British Medical Association's Concise Guide to Medicines and Drugs*. London: Dorling Kindersley, 2001.

House, Market., Hawthorn, Jan. *The A-Z of Medicinal Drugs: A Family Guide to Over-the-counter and Prescription Medicines*. Oxford: Oxford University Press, 2003.

Martin, Elizabeth. *Concise Medical Dictionary*. Oxford: Oxford University Press, 2007.

Clinical Knowledge Summaries (National Library for Health)—use Google and follow the links as required

CHAPTER
14

Making Treament Decisions

We hear about new treatments, new drugs, nutritional supplements, and alternative treatments all the time. Hardly a week goes by without a new treatment of some kind being reported in the news. We are bombarded in the market or pharmacy with signs and packaging for over-the-counter medicines and alternative treatments.

What can you believe? How can you decide what might be worth a try?

An important part of managing your own care is evaluating claims for new treatments so that you can make an informed decision about trying something new. Applying the steps outlined in chapter 2, *Becoming an Active Self-Manager* about action-planning would be very helpful here, to work through any decision in a systematic way, leaving room for review and change.

You need to get answers to some questions before you decide about any mainstream medical treatment you're offered, as well as complementary and alternative treatments.

1. **Where did you learn about this treatment?** Was it reported in a scientific journal, tabloid newspaper, print or TV advertisement, or a flyer you picked up somewhere? Did your doctor suggest it?

   It matters where information comes from. Results that are reported in a respected scientific journal are more believable than those you might see in the tabloids or on an advertising flyer. Results reported in scientific journals, such as *The British Medical Journal*, the *Lancet* or the *New England Journal of Medicine* are usually from research studies. These studies are closely reviewed for scientific integrity by other scientists, who are very careful about what they approve for publication. You need to know who has funded the research. Many alternative treatments and nutritional supplements have not been studied scientifically, so they are not as well represented in the scientific literature as medical treatments are. If this is the case, you need to be extra careful and critical about analysing what you read.

The Internet is a major resource for you because it can respond to new treatments very quickly, and is therefore a place to go for up-to-date information. Not everything on the Internet is correct or even safe so be cautious. Find the more reliable sites by looking for the author or sponsor of the site and the URL address. Addresses ending in .edu, .org, and .gov are generally more objective and reliable. These originate from universities, non-profit-making organisations, and governmental agencies. Some .com sites can also be good, but because they come from commercial or for-profit organisations, their information might be biased, as they are trying to promote or sell their own products. One good source for information about questionable treatments is Quackwatch, a non-profit-making corporation whose purpose is "to combat health-related frauds, myths, fads, and fallacies" (www.quackwatch.org). They also have other sites that are accessible from Quackwatch. Another good source is google scholar; it is quite scientifically orientated, but is useful because results are ordered according to the number of times a treatment is cited by other scientists as being useful or worthwhile. For more information on finding resources on the Internet and elsewhere, see chapter 3.

2. **Do research results come from studies on people like me?** In the past, many studies were done on college students, nurses, or white men. This has changed, but it is still important to find out if the people that got better were like you. Were they from the same age group? Did they have a similar lifestyle? Did they have the same health problems as you do? Were they the same sex and race? If the people aren't like you, the results may not be the same for you. Even if the subjects seem similar to you, the fact is that they *weren't* you, so all research data should be viewed as a guide to treatments, rather than as an absolute rule.

3. **Does the treatment suggest I change medicine or treatments I'm already having?** Would you have to stop taking another basic medicine because of dangerous interactions? You must talk to your prescribing doctor or pharmacist before making a change.

4. **Does the treatment suggest that I eat a diet that is not well-balanced for good health?** Does it eliminate any important nutrients or stress only a few nutrients that could be harmful to you? Maintaining a balanced diet is important for your overall health. Don't sacrifice important vitamins or else get them from another source if you change your eating habits. Also make sure that you're not putting excessive stress on your organs by concentrating on only a few nutrients.

5. **How can I find out about possible dangers?** Some treatments take a toll on your body. All treatments have side effects and possible risks. Discuss them with your doctor or your pharmacist. Only you can decide if the potential problems are worth the possible benefit, but you must have all the information in order to make that decision.

   Read labels and be aware of the language of selling. You might think that if something is "natural", it must be good for you. This may not be true. "Natural" isn't necessarily better just because it comes from a plant or animal. In the case of the powerful heart medication digitalis, which comes from the foxglove plant, it is "natural" but the dosage must be exact or it could be dangerous. Some treatments may be safe in small doses but dangerous in larger doses. Be careful to find out enough to make a proper decision. Words like "new" and "better" on labels are virtually meaningless, so be critical of what you read.

   Do some research about the company selling the product before you try it. There is no regulatory agency that is responsible for determining if what is listed on the label of a nutritional supplement is actually what's in the bottle, except in Germany. Supplements don't have the same safeguards as medications.

6. **Can I afford it?** What exactly will it cost you? Do you have the money to give a new treatment the time it needs to produce an improvement? Do the sums on paper as part of your action plan. It may be better not to start than to feel it is draining you financially and have to give it up.

7. **Am I willing to go to the trouble?** Analyse what you mean by "trouble" and consider the points as detailed and separate issues on your action plan. If you haven't, maybe you need to go back over these to get clear answers. What daily differences will the treatment make? Is your health strong enough to maintain this new regimen? Will you be able to handle it emotionally? Will it put a strain on your relationships at home and work?

8. **Do I have the necessary support in place?** Are there implications for the people you live with or your friends? Does your doctor support you? You are the one who decides, but after all, you and your doctor are partners, and you will need to keep them informed about your progress. Good communication while you are thinking about what to do helps them support you well.

9. **Can I be sure it's the treatment that made me feel better?** If you have done all your thinking and decided to go ahead, build in a review to your action plan. Try to identify what its actual effects are. People usually take up a generally healthier lifestyle when they begin a new treatment - could that be playing a part in the improvement? Have you started another medicine or treatment at the same time? Has the weather improved? Are you under less stress than before you started the treatment? What else might have affected your health? A woman who had just returned from a two-week stay at a spa in the tropics reported that her arthritis improved dramatically. But it's hard to attribute her improvement totally to the diet and supplements which made up "the treatment", when the warm weather, relaxation, and pampering may have had a lot to do with it!

When you can identify those changes which have got you closer to your goal, they can be built into future action plans, of course. Making well-informed and carefully reviewed choices about your treatment is an important and helpful part of active self-management and it is likely to reward your effort.

• • •

Suggested Further Reading

Egan, Gerard. *The Skilled Helper: A Problem-management and Opportunity Development Approach to Helping*, London: Thomson Learning, 2006.

Hargie, Owen. *A Handbook of Communication Skills*, 3rd Edition. London: Routledge, 2006.

Smith, Grainne. *Families, Carers and Professionals: Building Constructive Conversations*. West Sussex: John Wiley & Sons, 2007.

CHAPTER 15

Planning for the Future: Fears and Reality

People with chronic illnesses often worry about what will happen to them if their condition becomes really disabling. They fear that some time in the future they will have problems managing their day-to-day lives and their illness. They are afraid they may not be able to look after themselves and will be dependent on other people. They feel they could never bring themselves to accept help. They worry about money. Around all this, and the loss of freedom, there can be grief, anger and depression. The emotions people often have to tackle when dealing with a chronic condition make everything seem even more difficult even than it is—it is hard to think and act positively when you are sad and depressed. There can be low spots so low that nothing seems worth bothering with.

Perhaps you recognise some of the description above. When people start a self-management programme after diagnosis with a long-term condition, it can seem impossible to reach a place of acceptance, let alone happiness and even peace. But it has been done and you can do it too. Once you make the first step you can keep moving forward. Practical steps alter the perspective on the future, and the emotional landscape takes on a different shape and colour.

Action Planning to Gain Peace of Mind

Reading this book is a first step towards tackling fear, because one way people deal with fear of the future is to face it. Then they can take control and plan for it. They may very well never need to activate their plan, but there is reassurance in knowing that they will still be in control if the events they fear come to pass. The action planning method outlined in chapter 2, *Becoming an Active Self-Manager* can be applied to problems and goals at many levels—from "I want to go to the corner shop to buy a newspaper" to "I want to be content when I die". Making a start on dealing with the practicalities can make an impossible-sounding goal accessible.

The strength of action planning is that you break problems into "bite-size" portions. What may seem to be an insurmountable problem, your whole future, can be divided up into a set of much smaller issues, some of which can be dealt with right away. Making a change now or formulating a plan to deal with one part of your life can reshape your notion of your future. Problem-solving to sort out unforeseen difficulties is part of the process so as other things come up, you can deal with one at a time. Take it slowly and think carefully along the way about the realities of your situation and what you want to achieve.

Taking Control of Your Future

Action plans start with some sitting and thinking about what you want to do. The process of working out what you do want, begins with facing what you don't want, and that may mean confronting some bad feelings. If you want to, get some help around what you feel, but keep on with the action planning process in the meantime. Isolating your main practical issues from the general mass of worry is that first splendid step towards banishing the fear and taking control.

Action Planning for Day-to-Day Living

Issues around day-to-day living lend themselves very well to the action planning approach. The first thing to do is carefully evaluate what you can handle for yourself and what you may in future need help with—the everyday things like getting out of bed, bathing, dressing, preparing and eating your meals, cleaning the house, shopping, paying bills, and so on. Most people can do all these, even though they may have to do them slowly, with some modification or with some help from gadgets. If you fear you may eventually find one or more of these daily jobs no longer possible without help, explore the exact problem with the aim of working out what to do about it. For example, you may still be able to prepare and cook your meals, but you fear that you won't be able to walk well enough to get to the shops. Part of your condition may be that you faint without warning, and so for your safety you will need to have someone around all the time. Consider—

perhaps with a friend or family member to help bounce ideas off—what your symptoms lead you to fear in the future. Make a list of these, and don't worry about making a long list. It's better to have them all in front of you on paper, big and little, because from there, you can move on.

Action Planning for Day-to-Day Living

Examples

Can't go shopping	• Ask son/daughter to shop for me • Find a volunteer shopping service • Shop at a store that delivers • Ask neighbour to shop for me when she does her own shopping • Get meals-on-wheels
Can't be by myself	• Hire a full-time attendant • Move in with a relative • Get a local council emergency response system • Move to a residential care home • Move to a retirement community

When you have formulated and listed your problems, turn them around into statements of your goals. "I can't be by myself" turns into "I want someone to be near who can check I am all right". At that point, you are in a position to put into words as many options as you can think of—regardless of what you think at the moment is possible. Then you are ready to move on to step 3 and select the option that seems the most workable, acceptable, and within your budget. What you choose will depend upon your finances, the family, what is available in your area, other resources you can call on, and how well any of the options will in fact solve your problem. Sometimes, one choice would solve several problems. For instance, if you can't shop, can't be alone, and you really are beginning to welcome help with household chores, you might consider a retirement home to be a more than acceptable answer. It offers meals, regular house cleaning, and transport for errands and medical appointments. Choosing to adopt an option and turning it into an action plan which deals with all your stated anxieties is a different thing from thinking in despair "I can't cope, I'll have to give up and go into a home". If what you achieve is relief from many of the worries which undermine your happiness, you will have managed your situation without any loss of control and enabled yourself to move forward without regret.

Day-to-Day Living–Your Options

Staying at Home and Having Help Come to You

If you conclude that you need help with some activities, finding someone to help you in your home is less drastic than moving out and may be enough for quite a while. One option is pay privately for a home-help that you hire yourself. Another option for your list would be to find out what is being offered by your social services department. You have a right to ask for an assessment of your needs and this is an option in your action plan. This does not mean you have to accept the services they eventually offer, but it does give you a valuable starting point. The services offered are usually focused on making it possible for you to stay in your own home.

Home care services include personal care short of actual nursing. This might include helping you to get up and bathed in the morning and helping you to bed at night. It may be difficult to open yourself to so much help, but it will be a lot easier if you have considered the whole question in advance, well before you actually need it, and made a thoughtful choice from your options. It's self-management rather crisis management.

Services available for disabled people at home generally include adaptations to privately-owned or council-owned houses; equipment loan; meals on wheels; transport schemes; homecare services, advice and counselling; disabled parking badges, and usually, telephones for people who are housebound. In some parts of the UK, there will also be advice on state benefits. Some home care services also offer holiday schemes. If you arrive at the decision that you need this sort of help don't forget that you also need breaks, holidays and contact with your friends. These are part of your life and it is perfectly reasonable to ask for help to keep them going.

So, your first action plan if you are contemplating help at home either now or in the future, might be to find the number of your local authority social services department and ring them. Ask for a visit in your home or an appointment in the office, and approach the conversation with an open mind, to gather information to feed into your options. Finding out what's available doesn't commit you to anything.

Finding Partial Care or Staying at Home and Getting Some Care Outside

If one of the problems you identify is that you can't be alone, and the family member you live with is away from home during the day, explore the option of using an Age Concern or social services approved day centre. An advantage of this option is that day care centres are ideal places for you to find new friends and activities geared to your interests, while still being based at home.

Day Centres

Day centre services provided by local authorities and voluntary organisations can provide friendship and open doors to new activities or support. Some will be run directly by the local authority and others by local groups such as charities for older people, church groups or different ethnic minority groups. The organised activities may provide an opportunity for you to help as a volunteer, as well. As another resource, the other people you meet at a day centre will often have information of great use to you. You may have identified getting there and back as a problem in your action plan – you are likely to find day centres have their own transport services to take you to and from home.

Moving into Organized Care: Your Options Outside Your Home

Retirement Communities

Retirement Communities are becoming more popular and may be worth thinking about if you are over fifty, need little personal care and would like extra security and emergency response services. Communities are made up of owned or rented properties. There may be service charges around looking after buildings or gardens, and also for extra facilities, such as social activities or nursing care. There are waiting lists for retirement communities. If you want to go for this option, you should do the necessary registration as soon as you have made the decision, because many people find it an attractive option.

Sheltered Housing

Special Housing Associations provide sheltered housing. You live in your own small house or flat. You remain in control of how you run your life but a manager or warden sees you every day, and you have access to emergency support. Social events and meals are often arranged. Almshouses are available for some people on a low income or who have links with some of the craft guilds. Sheltered housing is not like residential care and the responsibility for your daily life will be your own.

Residential Care Homes

Residential care homes provide non-medical care and supervision for people who can't live alone. All homes, including Private Voluntary Homes, have to comply with the national minimum standards of the National Care Standards Commission. Look at the website www.doh.gov.uk/nssc/. Residential care is generally costly. A social services assessment would be needed for you to get help from the local authority. Homes vary in size. Services could include having all your meals provided; help with bathing and dressing; laundry; housekeeping; making medical appointments and help with taking medicines. You can use residential homes temporarily if you or your carers need a short break. This can be a chance to try out different local homes. Find out about the other residents of the home to see if they are likely to be good companions. Make sure the meals are to your liking and suit your ethnic background and any dietary needs. A good home will give you as much freedom as you want and support your independence.

Nursing Homes

Nursing homes provide care for very ill or disabled people who need skilled nursing care. Nearly all come under the National Care Standards Commission as Private Voluntary Homes. They are often used as a step between hospital care and home - someone who has had a stroke may be transferred from a hospital to a nursing home before going home. Many people spend a short time in a nursing home under Intermediate Care schemes. Qualified nurses provide specialised nursing care. Physiotherapists, occupational therapists and speech therapists also work in nursing homes. You would opt for a nursing home if you need a degree of regular personal help and nursing. Some nursing homes specialise in particular types of care or therapy. The hospital social work department can give you advice about selecting a nursing home if you are being discharged from hospital.

Incidentally, even if you are not of "retirement" age, many facilities accept daily visitors or residents as young as fifty, or younger if one of a couple is the minimum age. If you are a young person, a local authority social services disability section or Independent Living Centre should be able to direct you to a local facility appropriate for you.

Action Planning—Sorting Out Your Options

Using Your Consultants

You've got many possible consultants. You may well begin with the people immediately around you, family, friends or anyone you might feel able to ask to assist you. Clearly you will only speak about personal matters such as these to people you trust and to people to whom it won't be a burden. That means those closest to you may not be your best choice, and you may look for professional consultants, as you might also if you live alone. Some people find that talking with a sympathetic listener, either a professional counsellor or a sensible close friend or family member, is helpful. An objective listener can see options you may have overlooked. They can provide information, or another interpretation of a situation you haven't spotted. There may be someone from your church or religious community who is knowledgeable about situations such as yours. You might pay privately to talk to someone who can give you advice, or you may find it from social services and voluntary organisations. In practice, your desired arrangements for your care in the future are the central issue, and you will gather information and make arrangements with an assortment of individuals and organisations.

- Home carers—they have different titles in different authorities - are a vital source of information and a link to other services. Gradually the links between social service and health service nursing support are getting closer as administrative and budget systems to combine the services are increasingly established.
- Social workers from the local authority or the hospital social service department can help you with options for solving financial and living problems and telling you how to find what's available locally.
- Some social workers are trained in counselling disabled people and older people in relation to emotional and relationship problems that may be associated with your long-term condition.
- Health visitors can provide information to feed into your options.
- An occupational therapist can assess your daily living needs and suggest gadgets or ways of arranging your home to make life easier, and can help you formulate precisely what you need in a care facility.
- A Disabled Employment Advisor at the Local Job Centre can help with your working environment if you are employed.
- A solicitor specialising in the law for older people is worth consulting. They would help you set your financial affairs in order, to preserve your assets, to prepare a proper will, and perhaps to execute an enduring or temporary power of attorney for both health care and financial management. Consult chapter 11.

- Your local Citizens' Advice Bureau—CAB—and your local Law Society can supply you with the names of solicitors who offer free or low-cost services to older people. These solicitors are generally familiar with the laws applying to younger people with long-term conditions as well.
- Other resources to investigate include Age Concern day centres and other local organisations. Age Concern or the Citizens' Advice Bureau will know what's available in terms of welfare rights. They often have listings of local services, both professional and voluntary. It's best to go through a list of this sort, because the staff will have been vetted.
- You can also get expert advice from Independent Welfare Rights Advice agencies and in local authority welfare rights departments.

Who Not to Consult!

It's worth using lists of consultants from your local authority, for example, or from a voluntary organisation, if you will need to invite visitors or helpers you don't know into your house, because you have the security of knowing the staff have been screened by the police.

Be very careful with advice from somebody who has something to sell you. There are many people whose solution to your problem just happens to be whatever they're selling—funeral insurance policies, special and expensive furniture, "sunshine cruises," special magazines, or health foods with magical curative properties. Of course you will approach people whose product you want to buy, but in general, research the area first, and don't have people into your home unless you have a strong and confident person to sit with you while you talk—even if you are strong and confident yourself. And don't sign anything there and then! Take time to think.

The list of possible living arrangements above can be used to support your search for information as you develop a vision of and some plans for your future.

Action Planning to Pay for Care

When you list the options for the action plan you are making, in case you should eventually need more care, put down everything you can think of. Deal with each anxiety and objection which comes up as a separate issue and write it down as a whole sentence. "If I go away from here, I'm afraid I won't see my friends any more." "I worry that I haven't got enough money to pay nursing home fees." Money features large amongst most people's anxieties.

As with any other action plan, there is a stage of gathering information. For example, you may need to start small, by having as one action plan to look up the numbers and ring the care homes you know about. You may ask them for their literature, or you could simply ask what it costs to stay there for a month. Keep a proper written list of the facts, and eventually, a whole file of the information you gather. You may at the same time plan to find out where you could get financial help from, so another action plan could be a call to the local Social Services department to ask for an assessment of your needs, and for all the information they can give you about state benefits or other assistance. The good thing about doing this is that when you know more, you fear less. You stop feeling so reluctant to do something when you know better what you might do.

Make sure you have the financial facts in black and white in front of you, and get someone you trust to help you read the figures, do the sums and see what's possible.

Consider the possible costs of equipment and services, if your plan is to stay at home. Consider purchase or rent costs if you plan to move to another room, flat, house or community, and the costs of extra services provided in those places. You will also be gathering facts about your own income, savings, assets, the value of your house, and you will have explored the help available to you from the social services. The information you have gathered about possible living arrangements can be used alongside your knowledge of the facts of your money, to develop a vision of and plans for your future.

Of course, no decision-taking is ever a tidy set of logical steps, but as you work on the detail of your options and assemble concrete information about what you might do if eventually you can't look after yourself, it may be that a new view of your future will emerge.

Action Planning to Accept Loss

People with a chronic, disabling health problem experience loss. There may have been a gradual development and then diagnosis of chronic disease. Slowly the realisation of the implications follows. There may be actual changes in lifestyle. People begin to face what they imagine to be their future, which can look frightening. There are two necessary overall tasks. The first is to accept the losses and maximise the life choices available, via action planning round symptom self-management. The second is to deal with fear of the future, including issues with dying and death. The tasks of course overlap but as with other areas of your life, action planning can help to untangle some of the strands. The rest of the chapter looks at options for sorting some emotional strands, and at some practical activities for taking control around the uncertainties of dying as far as anyone can.

The losses people experience can include independence, self-esteem and confidence. They lose elements of the lifestyle they knew and cherished. Positive self-image may be lost, if physical appearance and activities have had to change. Fear of the future can include fear of further losses, physically, financially and emotionally. People fear the loss of independence and privacy that may accompany being helped with daily activities. They fear deeply that people will no longer love them, even to the extent of being abandoned by family members who might have helped. These are major issues, not the less so because almost everybody has to face them sooner or later.

When we experience any kind of a loss, small and trivial or large and life-changing, we go through an emotional process of grieving and coming to terms with it. Elizabeth Kübler-Ross, who has written extensively about this process, describes the stages of grief. First, she says, there is shock, when people feel both a mental and a physical reaction to the initial recognition of the loss. Next, denial, when people tell themselves, “No, it can’t be true”, and act for a time as if it were not true. Then there is a stage of anger, “why me?” searching for someone or something to blame—“if the doctor had diagnosed it early enough I’d have been cured”, or “the job caused me too much stress”. She sees the next stage as bargaining, when people say to themselves or someone else, or God, “I’ll never smoke again”, or “I’ll follow my treatment regimen absolutely to the letter”, or “I’ll go to church every Sunday, if only I can get over this”. When the real awareness sets in, and people confront the truth, they experience deep feelings of sadness and hopelessness. These feelings can turn to depression, if people get stuck in them. Finally, people reach acceptance, when they can deal with what has happened and make up their minds to do what they have to do. At this point, many people discover renewed pleasure in their life.

People don’t pass through these stages in a straight line. Stages overlap and recur. There tend to be several, or even many, flip-flops back and forth between them. Although analyses like these are useful to know, since they suggest that there is a path through a very difficult period of our lives, they can make us feel as though we “ought” to have “got through that stage by now”. There is no one route and no fixed timescale. If you have experienced some or all of these stages since you became ill, don’t be discouraged if you find yourself angry or depressed again, when you thought you had reached acceptance. You are not moving backwards—it's much more like a spiral, where people steadily move "up" but keep on having to go over similar ground. Your aim in "working on your feelings", if you choose to, is to help yourself move on through your own journey without getting stuck.

The feelings people with chronic conditions face often come from a basic dilemma. "Yes, I need help. No, I don't want it. Now what?" It can be very frustrating to be caught like this. We generally recognise it if we feel "frustrated" but the term is not much help when it comes to dealing with underlying feelings, because all it means is that we feel prevented from what doing what we want. Sometimes people move from "frustration" to "depression" and remain stuck, without being clear what feelings are churning around underneath the surface. It's worth spending some time familiarising yourself with what your underlying feelings are, if you feel like this, because that gradually allows movement towards acceptance.

It can be helpful to think of an emotion, which is your feeling getting moving and wanting to be expressed, as if it were a very small child wanting your attention. They call you, they tug your clothes, they keep on at you and just won't stop. They appear unreasonable – to an adult who has "important adult stuff" to do. They go on and on until, exasperated, you look at them, ask them what's the matter, and listen to the answer. You pay them proper attention and they go away and leave you in peace. Anger, grief, regret, sadness and other feelings all do this. They really want to be noticed and they nag away at you. Like a busy parent with a child, you say, "In a minute!" .You've got your life to lead, jobs to do, people to see - you haven't got time to sit down and notice how cross or miserable you feel. Quite likely you don't even admit the feelings are there. So you ignore them, and in the end, they go off silently, like a child might. The problem is not solved, however, just hidden. The good news is that once feelings have been noticed, properly, by your body and your mind, they will let you be. Counselling and other therapies work on this sort of idea, in that they allow you to look properly at what you have pushed away. Healing starts from "looking properly" and acknowledging the feelings, because after that, people don't stay stuck and are free to move on with their lives.

One of the problems that may need solving in your action plan is that people sometimes think it is self-indulgent or weak to focus on feelings. Not true—it takes strength to take the first step towards noticing them. Other people might think that acknowledging a feeling would give it power and it could then overwhelm them. People think "If I start to cry, I'll never stop" and they prefer not to "lose control". The clever thing about the body is that it gets tired, so you do stop crying. You can't sustain furious anger for long if you are punching a cushion. Afterwards, you find the feeling has lost some of its power over you, as the tug of that unregarded emotion causes less agitation of your mind. Our society does not generally allow us to express extreme emotions. From childhood both sexes are encouraged not to cry. On the whole, we don't raise our voices in the presence of other people. We often live so close to other people that we have no opportunity to wail our grief or shout our anger. Our pain can make other people uncomfortable. Clearly if we all carried on like the imagined child above, yelling until we were noticed, it would be an unruly society. However, it becomes necessary for individuals to work out ways of dealing with their own emotional upheavals in a healthy, if private, manner.

This is where you can use your mind to manage your emotional symptoms. Use an adapted action plan to sort out what your feelings are and decide on some steps to release them. There are options for methods of working on what you feel. One option is to sit still, alone, regularly, and contemplate as honestly as possible. If feelings come up in an emotional response like tears, let them, with confidence that they will weaken and go away if you let them come. Another option is to write. Many people find great solace in putting their feelings down on paper. Some may write in their journal, some may write a poem or a story, or a letter which is not intended for sending. If writing is hard, talking onto an audiotape is a good substitute. Another option is to talk to a friend—sometimes difficult because neither you nor your friend wants to upset the other, but a trusted friend can be of great help as a listener. A fourth option is to find professional counselling, someone who is trained to be sympathetic but uninvolved, who does not give advice or comfort, but just lets you hear what you say—in other words, enables you to pay proper attention with your mind to your feelings. When you consider which option to pick, there may be determining factors in your situation – not enough privacy, not enough money, or simply that you're not ready to do this yet. Take these into account as you decide what to do. If you are attracted to the idea of counselling, your local authority social services or a support group for people with your condition might be able to refer you to an appropriate counsellor. Look in Yellow Pages under the listing "social service organisations," or on the Internet, or ask one of your consultants. Once again, you may find there is financial help for those who need it.

Action Planning to Face Fear of Death

What people often fear about death is dying. Some things about dying cannot be known until they happen and our fear is perhaps more to do with the unknown, than of death itself. "What will it be like?" "Will it be painful?" There is a different set of questions around "What will happen to me when I die?" which are addressed by many people through a religious or spiritual search. This early part of this chapter looks at how modified action planning can be used to help with feelings about living with a chronic illness. This section suggests how you might choose to untangle and clarify some of your feelings about dying. Action planning around practical matters can reduce the scale of the unknown and make it more manageable.

Nurses who care for the dying observe that nearly everybody is ready to die when the time comes. Something in the process which the living cannot know changes people's ordinary consciousness, which experiences resistance to dying, to a state of mind that can accept it. Most people just "slip away," with the transition between the state of living and no-longer-living hardly identifiable. People who have lived through a "near-death experience", in that their bodies showed the lack of vital signs suggesting clinical death, say that they felt peaceful and clear, and were not frightened.

However, a person approaching death may sometimes feel lonely and abandoned. Perhaps the friends and family of someone who is dying can't deal with their own emotions. They are anxious not to make the situation "worse" by breaking down. The acknowledgment that a person is dying can be difficult, and indeed no-one can be sure exactly what will happen, or when, and that uncertainty can be hard to deal with. Embarrassment can lead to superficial chitchat, broken by long awkward silences. Friends and family may deliberately avoid the dying person's company. This can be puzzling and hurtful to the dying person, who needs companionship and solace. One of the benefits of action plans is that while you are working on them, you will be talking about your feelings about your death, in the context of practical arrangements. This may make it easier for you and the people round you to share your views. People who are reluctant to initiate such a conversation may appreciate your bringing it up. You can use the discussion around your plans to sort out the extent of the help you may need and ask for, and how much those around you are able and willing to give. You can avoid misunderstandings.

If you've spoken to a counsellor about your feelings around being ill, it's likely the subject of dying and death will have come up. It's an option to find a counsellor if you have more to explore than your friends or family can cope with. Also, if you cannot turn to close family or friends you may be able to find a "case manager" through your local social services or your hospital social services departments. They can organise community resources to help you.

Thinking ahead in terms of your options, while you are fit to plan, can reduce difficulty in the future. It can certainly reduce your fear or anxiety now. People find they can begin to come to terms with their eventual death by taking positive steps to prepare for it. Making practical plans, and talking them over as you go, can clear the air with people around you, too. If the plans need to be put into effect, the practical arrangements and some of the emotional issues will have been dealt with. Have a look at chapter 9 *Communicating* and chapter 11, *Making Your Wishes Known.*

Action Planning for Dying and Death

Consider and decide where you would want to be—at home, in a hospice or in hospital—during your last days and hours, and who should be with you. Make a will. Even if your estate is a small one you may want to find out and plan in advance how the disposal of it could affect your heirs and to make it explicit what should happen to it. Make arrangements for your funeral. There are prepaid "future need" funeral plans available. Make an Enduring Power of Attorney for health care, and an Enduring Power of Attorney for your financial affairs. Assemble details of bank and credit card accounts, insurance policies, savings, your safe deposit box and keys. Some shops stock a personal file with headings to guide your filing of all the documentation necessary to getting your affairs in order. Gather your paperwork and file it together to enable your executors to find everything. As you pay your debts and settle your affairs, you are in a position to finish your "business" in the world, mend your relationships and say what needs to be said to those who need to hear it.

Active Self-Management and Taking Control

This chapter suggests taking control of as much as you can of your future by re-formulating your situation in small steps which are manageable for you. It suggests extending the skills of active self-management in your daily life into planning for your care and your death in the future, in order to release you from worry and fear, allowing you freedom to enjoy your life today to the full. When we find "the courage to change the things we can", then perhaps we are closer to the "serenity to accept the things we cannot". Looking at what you want to do, and deciding what first step to take, provides a strong foundation for making decisions yourself. If you are facing an uncertain future, but have taken necessary decisions before they are needed, you are taking control and keeping the right to make your own decisions. Action planning enables systematic and careful consideration of all the options, so that when you have changed what you can change, your wise acceptance of things you can't allows the people around you to respect your decisions. It frees them to give you the help you have chosen. If you do reach a situation where you have to accept help, you will have done so from a position of strength. Your dignity is safeguarded by your forethought and use of choice.

• • •

Suggested Further Reading

Disability Rights Handbook. This is published each year by the Disability Alliance. For details phone 020 7247 8776.

.Callahan, Maggie, and Patricia Kelley. *Final Gifts: Understanding the Special Awareness, Needs, and Communications of the Dying.* New York: Bantam Books, 1997.

Copeland, Mary Ellen, and Wayne London. *The Depression Workbook: A Guide for Living with Depression and Manic Depression.* Oakland, Calif.: New Harbinger Publications, 1992.

Gilbert, Paul. *Overcoming Depression.* Constable Robinson, 2000.

Lewinsohn, Peter M., editor. *Control Your Depression.* Simon & Schuster, 1992.

Carter, Roselynn,, Lynn, Joanne., Harrold, Joan., *Handbook for Mortals: Guidance for People Facing Serious Illness.* Oxford: Oxford University Press, 2001.

Whybrow, Ruth. *Caring for Elderly Parents.* Crossroads Publishers, 1996.

CHAPTER 16

Helpful Hints

People with long-term conditions sometimes face practical problems in their everyday life. They solve them creatively and ingeniously, often with a very minor adjustment to what's available. In a small way, they have applied an action plan – what's my problem, what's my goal, what are my options, do they work, what's my new problem? And then rewarded themselves with the satisfaction of a more manageable life! You have probably solved many of your daily problems too. Perhaps these hints, gathered from others facing similar problems, will activate your problem-solving skills even further. Not everything works for everyone. Use what is helpful.

First big hint—PACE YOURSELF. Build timing into your action-planning and do as you have planned. You can modify the plan next time as you are able to do more.

Waking Up

- Try some stretching and strengthening exercises while you are still in bed.
- Consider an electric mattress pad if extra heat will help loosen morning stiffness.
- Get a clock radio and have music to wake you instead of an alarm. If your radio can wake you with a tape or CD function, pre-record your own "pep-talk".
- A duvet can replace a bedspread and is easy to pull up.

- Straighten half your bedclothes while you are still in it and can reach. Then get out of the unmade side.
- Do some of your dressing sitting on the edge of your bed before you get up. Leave the clothes within reach of your bed the night before.
- Keep a walking stick or chair next to your bed to help pull yourself out of bed in the morning.

Bathing

- If you find standing in a shower or sitting down in the bath difficult, get a bath stool. It is waterproof and fits in the bath. You can sit while you bathe.
- Replace shower heads or bath taps with a hand-held sprayer unit.
- If you are feeling weak, a "sponge bath" can be taken in place of a full bath and can be a lot less taxing. Don't shower if you are at home alone.
- Using a long, absorbent, cotton terry robe cuts out the effort of drying with a towel.
- Soap on a rope lets you use soap with one hand, and keeps it from falling.
- A liquid soap dispenser may be easier to use than a bar of soap.
- Replace difficult twist tops on shampoo or lotions with pump tops.
- A shower caddy keeps bathing supplies within easy reach.
- Use non-skid safety strips or a rubber bath mat in the bath or shower.
- Consider having grab bars installed in your bath or shower to reduce the risk of falling.
- Get a long-handled sponge or brush.

- Suctioned soap holders make it possible to soap yourself without grasping the soap or needing to use two hands.

Looking after Your Teeth

- Suctioned brushes are useful for cleaning dentures with one hand.
- Electric toothbrushes make brushing easier.
- Get a dental-floss holder if flossing is difficult with two hands.
- Look for toothpaste in pumps rather than tubes. The heel of one hand can press the pump.
- Look for special long or curved handled toothbrushes.
- Toothbrush handles can be made easier to grasp by wrapping a small sponge or foam hair curler around them.

Hygiene

- Ask family members to fold the end of the toilet paper into a "V" to make it easier to get hold of.
- Hand-held female urinals available from travel supply companies make it possible for a woman to urinate standing up.
- Women who sometimes accidentally pass urine find small panty liners or sanitary pads with adhesive backs helpful.
- If you use sanitary towels, you can keep the genital area clean using a squeeze bottle of water kept by the toilet. These bottles can be found with a variety of spray nozzles.
- If you find tampons difficult to remove you might try winding the tampon string round a pencil and gently pulling it with both hands. Some brands have looped strings.
- Have a grab bar or safety frame installed next to the toilet. A stable free-standing towel rack next to the toilet can also help you when getting off the toilet.

Grooming

- A small sponge around the handle of a razor or an eyeliner pencil can make them easier to grasp.
- You can reach your hair more easily with long-handled combs and brushes.

- Shaving or applying make-up is easier if you have a mirror set low enough for you to sit down.
- Talk to your hairdresser about a style that's easy to maintain. Cut out the need for rollers and hairdryers.
- If you have respiratory problems, switch to non-aerosol toiletries. You can get liquid hair dressings and roll-on deodorants.
- You can get unscented and hypoallergenic toiletries.

Dressing

- Spend some time problem-solving around your clothes storage, to organise drawers so that you can reach your clothes without strain.
- Lower the rail in your wardrobe or get a wardrobe organiser to help you reach your clothes.
- It is safer and easier to pull underpants and trousers up when lying on the bed.
- Shop for clothes with dressing in mind. Look for easy-to-reach fasteners, front openings, and elastic waistbands loose enough to be pulled over the hips.
- Look for clothes with Velcro or elastic instead of buttons.
- Replace the buttons on your garments with Velcro. Move the buttons to the top part of the opening for decoration.
- Bras can be fastened in front and then turned around and pulled into place, or buy front-opening bras.
- Avoid tight belts, bras or girdles which limit how far and how easily you can breathe in.

- Avoid tight neck bands. Ties should be loose or replaced with a loosely tied scarf.
- Braces might be easier to manage and more comfortable than a belt.
- Dusting powder on the thighs makes pulling on tights easier.
- Trousers and socks may be easier to manage than struggling into tights.
- Put rings or loops on zip fasteners to make it easier to pull zips.
- If hot or cold temperatures bother you, you may find cotton underclothing more comfortable than synthetic.
- Use a bent coat hanger to help with retrieving clothes that are out of reach.
- Get a long-handled shoehorn.
- Slip-on shoes are easier than tying laces.
- Convert lace-up shoes to slip-ons with elastic shoelaces.
- When shopping for clothes, take a tape measure with you that is marked with your measurements. By measuring the garments, you may not have to try on so many before you buy.
- Choose trousers or women's skirts with pockets, and carry money, driver's licence, and so on, in the pockets instead of carrying a large, heavy handbag. There are "travel" gilets and waistcoats available with several secure pockets.
- Avoid socks or stockings with elastic bands or garters, which may bind the leg and restrict circulation.
- Dress in layers so you can adjust quickly to changes in temperature. Use good underwear to provide heat without weight.

Getting Around

- Lead with your stronger leg when going up stairs. Lead with your weaker leg when going down.
- Remove all loose rugs—they can cause falls.

- Taking off the doors can make doorways wide enough to let you move freely with a wheelchair, a walking aid or other equipment.
- Consider installing stair rails on both sides of the stairway to increase safety.
- A small ramp can replace a couple of stairs at the entrance to your home or elsewhere. Be careful of building regulations, though!
- Carry a folding walking chair seat with you when you go out. You can lean on it or sit down when you need to.
- Place a chair or table near the top of stairs to lean or sit on when you reach the top.
- For a job that takes effort, lift or carry while breathing out through pursed lips. Rest and breathe in through your nose. Keep this up till you have finished.
- Look for a walker that has a large basket in front and a small bench seat to sit on when you get tired.
- Consider installing a mechanical lift chair on your stairs.

Doing Household Chores

- Get a small serving trolley. As you do the household chores, use the trolley to carry your supplies or things that need to be put away.
- Have a trolley upstairs and downstairs.
- Keep a set of cleaning supplies in each area where they are to be used to avoid carrying them around.
- Plan your chores so that you go in a circle, rather than back and forth.
- Reachers can retrieve things from hard-to-reach places. You can buy them from Boots and most other medical supply shops.
- A magnet tied to a string can help pick up drawing pins, hairpins, and so on. It will stick to your trolley, refrigerator or washing machine for storage.

- Long-handled sponges are good for hard-to-reach areas such as your bath.
- To clean your bathtub, sit on a low stool next to the tub and use a long-handled sponge.
- Clean the bath when you are still in it. Then rinse both you and it.
- Consider a battery-powered "scrubber" for bathtub, sink, and so on.
- Get a long-handled dustpan and a small broom for dry spills.
- Foam floor mats can be placed where you may need to stand often, such as at the sink, ironing board, or telephone. They can reduce foot and ankle pain and low back pain.
- Use an adjustable-height ironing board so that you can sit down while ironing.
- Divide the ironing pile into "urgent and important", "important but not urgent", "not important and/not urgent" (do these need ironing at all?)—and do a small amount at a time.
- Small items such as socks or underwear can be washed in laundry bags to avoid having to search in the washer or dryer.
- If lifting heavy detergent boxes is difficult, have someone pour some into a small container, or put a large container on the floor and use a scoop.
- Use gravity to get clothes out of the dryer or front-loading washer. Put a basket under the door and scoop the clothes into it with a reacher or stick.
- Try old-fashioned push-on clothes pegs rather than ones you have to pinch.
- Fitted bottom sheets are difficult to put on the bed, slit one corner and fasten with a tie.
- Use a large, wide spatula to tuck in sheets.
- Use a vacuum cleaner with disposable bags; remove the bag straight into a binbag if you dust bothers you.
- A small, battery-powered hand vacuum cleaner is easy to use for small areas and can be kept on your trolley.

- Avoid sweeping and dusting if you have breathing problems. If you feel you must do it, wrap the working end of the broom or mop with a damp cloth.
- Wear a mask against dust.
- A damp cloth is good for dusting. For wooden surfaces, get a roll of paper towels and a bottle of lemon oil. Put a few dots of oil on each towel, use and throw away.
- People with respiratory problems should not use aerosol cleaning products.
- Avoid substances that can vapourise, such as mothballs, solvents, and kerosene.
- Ventilate your rooms with fresh air all the time.
- Put lockable castors on furniture you need to move for cleaning.
- Don't dismiss decorating your house as impossible without considering applying action-planning, to break it down into manageable sections.

Cooking, Eating and Kitchen Stuff

- Use a microwave oven to save time and energy.
- Replace the twist-ties on bread or other foods with plastic clips.
- Avoid lifting heavy pots of food along with the water they were cooked in. Put food in a basket to lower into the water for cooking, or get a spaghetti cooker with holes in. Lift the basket out to drain food. Someone else can drain the pot later, or you can ladle the water out.
- Ask family members not to close jars too tightly. A jar opener can be mounted under a work-surface, or you can get a rubber disk to help you open jars.
- Try to replace heavy pots and pans with a weight you can manage.
- Don't try to get everything done at once. Divide up your jobs—clean the top shelf of the refrigerator today and the bottom shelf tomorrow.

- Plan your meals when you are not hungry and not tired. You need to organise for the Balance of Good Health—see chapter 12, *Healthy Eating*—and you can't do that at the last moment when you're starving.
- Use offers of help to get vegetables peeled and cut up, for later or for freezing.
- Have a water container that has a tap near the bottom so that you won't have to lift a whole bottle to fill your drinking glass.
- Cook double or triple quantities of the recipe. Freeze the extra portions in meal-sized containers. In a microwave, they can be easily thawed and heated without drying out.
- Try a slow-cooker which lets you prepare while you're not tired. A pressure cooker can help too.
- Use an extractor fan when cooking, especially if you have respiratory problems.
- A small, portable fan can help you overcome shortness of breath or cool you off in a warm kitchen. Some are battery-powered and can clip on to a shelf.
- Use your trolley when tidying up after a meal. Gather all the items that need to go into the refrigerator, and then sit down with the trolley and put them away all at once.
- Put your most-used pots and pans back on the cooker and leave them there.
- Instead of putting dishes and cutlery away, maybe reset the table for the next meal.
- Use disposable foil tins to help at the cleaning up stage.
- Line pans with aluminium foil
- Buy non-stick pans.
- Try a serving dish with spikes sticking up that will hold meat firmly in place while you cut it. If necessary, you will be able to carve meat with one hand.
- When you buy kitchen appliances, look for pushbuttons or levers you find easy to use.

- Put flour and sugar in handy containers so that you won't have to lift the heavy bags.
- Oven gloves let you lift hot pans with both hands.
- A pizza wheel can cut it easily!
- A small food processor can make grating, chopping, or slicing easier.

- Wheeled stools in the kitchen will make work easier, either to sit on at a work surface or low enough help you get to lower shelves.
- Use a pizza cutter to cut your food into bite-size pieces.
- Use a scoop dish with a non-skid bottom to avoid pushing food off the plate.

Entertaining

- Buffets are easy. Let guests serve themselves.
- Use disposable plates and utensils.
- Plan a potluck rather than doing it all yourself.
- Dessert potlucks are especially popular.
- Buy two tickets for an event and ask a friend.

Remembering to Take Medicines

- A pillbox with a separate compartment for each day of the week is useful. A pillbox can be home-made out of an egg carton or bought at your local chemist.
- Some electronic pillboxes can be programmed to "beep" you when it's time to take your medicine.
- Combine medicine taking with a normal, daily habit, such as brushing your teeth. Put your pills next to the things you use for that activity, such as a toothbrush, making sure your medicines are out of the reach of children.

- When you get a prescription, work out how long it will last and mark the time to re-order on a calendar. This may save you from running out at a weekend or holiday.
- Put a reminder note on the bathroom mirror, the refrigerator door, the coffee maker, the television, or some other conspicuous place.
- Make a medicine chart containing each medicine you are taking and when you take it. Tick off each medicine as you take it noting the time and date.
- Buy a "medicines organiser" at the chemist. This container separates pills according to the time of day they should be taken. You fill the organiser once a week so that all your pills are ready to take at the proper time. A quick glance at the organiser lets you know if you have missed any doses and prevents double dosing.
- Get a watch that can be set to beep at pill-taking time.
- Ask other family or household members to help remind you to take your medicines.
- If you're travelling, put a note in your luggage reminding you to pack your pills.
- Take an extra prescription in your carry-on luggage in case you lose your pills or your luggage.

Shopping

- Do it little and often.
- Build in a rest part of the way through.
- Make it sociable and meet a friend.
- If you have a computer, you can shop on the Internet.
- Find grocery shops and chemists or pharmacies who will deliver to your home.
- At the supermarket check out always ask for help with packing.
- Balance the bags and keep them small.

- Pack your fresh, chilled and frozen foods items in separate bags so that you can unpack and put away in stages when you get home.
- Some shopping centres now offer shopability schemes with powered wheelchairs equipped with shopping trolleys. Find out how you can be taught how to use them.
- Use offers of help to get shopping done for you.
- Explore local or community offers to shop for you.
- Mail-order catalogues offer some of the things you would want, and are fun to look through.

Going Out

- Get assertive about exposure to other people's tobacco smoke. You have a right to breathe smoke-free air. Ask smokers politely but clearly to stop.
- Wash your hands well when you get home. Colds and other diseases are often spread by touch.
- Before going out, prepare for your return home. Lay out your comfortable clothes and slippers, leave a drink in a handy thermos, set out what you will need for your evening meal. Coming in will be a pleasure.
- If you don't already have one, ask your social services department about getting a disabled parking permit. Even if you don't drive, a friend can use this when you go out together.
- If you fill the petrol tank, try to position yourself upwind so that you don't breathe in the fumes.
- When shopping for a new car, look for easily-opened doors and easily-adjusted seats. Attach a loop to the inside door handle of your car to make it easier to pull it closed.
- Get plastic extenders that make seat belts easier to get hold of if they go back behind your shoulder.
- Wide-angle rear-view mirrors allow you to see better without hurting your neck.

- A back support device can make a car seat more comfortable.
- Consider having a mobile phone if you haven't already.

Gardening

- Use a cooker timer or an alarm clock to remind you to stop when you planned.
- A sit-in, motorised lawnmower can be a real morale booster.
- Find lightweight, easy-to-handle tools.
- Use a folding stool or one with wheels. There are wheeled stools especially for gardening, with a tool storage area under the seat.
- Many tools can be purchased with a long handle, or you can have a short handle replaced with a long one.
- Use raised beds so that you can sit on the edge and reach without bending.

Enjoying Recreation and Leisure

- Get to know your neighbours.
- Somewhere near you there is someone who needs your friendship and help. Look for these opportunities.
- Set up a telephone network with friends. Apart from a good gossip, these friends might be able to help in an emergency.
- Arrange a signal, such as a pulled-down blind at night, to let your neighbours know you are all right.
- Home computers and digital television services are becoming more affordable.
- You can play long-distance board games by email.
- You can play some games over the phone.
- Your computer can introduce you to other people through chat rooms and by e-mail. Be cautious!

- Learn to use your computer in an adult education class in your local community. This can be a way of meeting interesting people.
- Join an art class.
- If you like to paint at home, consider watercolours. They are lightweight, odourless, and dry quickly. You don't need to be good at it to enjoy it.
- The Open College and the Open University offer adult education classes through television or correspondence.
- If your previous hobbies are too demanding, try scaling them down. Focus on houseplants or a window box or an indoor herb garden, rather than a whole garden.
- An embroidery frame and stand will allow you to do needlework without having to use your hands to stabilise the piece you are working on.
- Self-threading needles are available at fabric shops and through catalogues. Ask a relative to give you threaded needles for your birthday.

Travelling

- Enjoy the planning as well as the travelling.
- Ask your doctor about your tolerance to altitude and cabin air pressures before you travel by air. Be aware of the altitude of your destination.
- Use all the help the airline or train company can offer you—find out what's available in your action planning stage.
- You can arrange in advance with airlines for a wheelchair, special boarding and seating, or special meals. Confirm the arrangements at least forty-eight hours before your flight.
- Travel light. Get suitcases with well spaced wheels, or get a rolling luggage rack.
- Find out if there is a travel agent in your area who specialises in travel for people with physical limitations.

- Instead of a handbag, use a waistcoat with lots of pockets.
- Do ankle and leg exercises to keep the blood flowing in your legs and feet, and to avoid clots.
- When you fly, drink enough water and avoid offers of alcohol.
- Explore travellers' gadgets in mail order catalogues and travel shops. Nearly everything anyone could need is marketed!

Getting Sleep

- Go to bed in stages so that you arrive relaxed, not worn out. Put on your nightclothes and then relax by reading or watching television for a little while.
- Have a telephone and a light in easy reach.
- Attach emergency numbers to the phone, or use a phone with an auto-dial feature.
- A night-light will help prevent falls or feeling disorientated in the dark.
- Keep a torch near the bed for emergencies.
- Keep spare spectacles by the bed.
- Bedtime is often a good time to do some gentle muscle-relaxation exercises.

Keeping Warm

- Heating pads come in many shapes and sizes, to fit just about any part of your body.
- Soak stiff, sore hands or feet in warm water.
- Thermoelastic gloves are good for warming. They are available at some chemists. Thermoelastic products are also available for knees and elbows.
- Electric blankets and electric mattress pads are lightweight and warm.

- Sleeping inside a sleeping bag placed under a blanket will help to keep you warm.
- Consider wearing long underwear. It comes in many colours and styles. Silk is luxurious!
- A large shawl is good for the occasional shivers, and much easier to put on and take off then a sweater.
- Avoid really cold places if you have respiratory problems.

• • •

Suggested Further Reading

Biegel, David E., Eva Kahana, and May Wykle. *Family Caregiving Across the Lifespan.* Sage Publications Inc., 1994.

You can also get ideas about helpful equipment from a Disabled Living Centre. There are many centres across the UK and their website has addresses and phone numbers: www.dlcc.org.uk

Index

Notes

Notes

Notes

Notes